Healthcare Innovation Success

Penny Kechagioglou

Healthcare Innovation Success

Learning from Organisational Experience

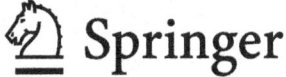

Penny Kechagioglou
Warwick Business School
University of Warwick
Coventry, UK

ISBN 978-3-031-28352-9 ISBN 978-3-031-28353-6 (eBook)
https://doi.org/10.1007/978-3-031-28353-6

© The Editor(s) (if applicable) and The Author(s), under exclusive license to
Springer Nature Switzerland AG 2023
This work is subject to copyright. All rights are solely and exclusively licensed by the Publisher, whether the whole or part of the material is concerned, specifically the rights of translation, reprinting, reuse of illustrations, recitation, broadcasting, reproduction on microfilms or in any other physical way, and transmission or information storage and retrieval, electronic adaptation, computer software, or by similar or dissimilar methodology now known or hereafter developed.
The use of general descriptive names, registered names, trademarks, service marks, etc. in this publication does not imply, even in the absence of a specific statement, that such names are exempt from the relevant protective laws and regulations and therefore free for general use.
The publisher, the authors, and the editors are safe to assume that the advice and information in this book are believed to be true and accurate at the date of publication. Neither the publisher nor the authors or the editors give a warranty, expressed or implied, with respect to the material contained herein or for any errors or omissions that may have been made. The publisher remains neutral with regard to jurisdictional claims in published maps and institutional affiliations.

This Springer imprint is published by the registered company Springer Nature Switzerland AG
The registered company address is: Gewerbestrasse 11, 6330 Cham, Switzerland

Preface

For all of us who work in healthcare, we can recognise clinical research as being a core activity in everything we do and with clear processes to guide us through it. Across the globe, clinical research has led to the discovery of new medications for diseases and to service changes leading to better healthcare. But when it comes to innovation in healthcare, the journey from an idea to the implementation has no clear path and often good ideas do not translate into practice change. Healthcare innovation involves the design of new services and products to meet healthcare needs or the improvement of existing services and is often initiated by front line clinical innovators, who are committed to finding solutions to common healthcare problems. For innovations to become sustained, they need to pass some essential stages such as adoption, diffusion and implementation and the problem with healthcare innovations is that they often stall at the adoption stage.

Leadership within healthcare organizations is considered to be a key driver for all stages of innovation, from ideation to adoption, diffusion, implementation and innovation sustainability. The role of individual and organizational leadership in driving the different stages of innovation needs to be further explored and understood so that systems and frameworks are put in place to enable innovation success. In the current volatile, competitive and unpredictable external environment, healthcare organizations need to think and operate differently and more innovatively, in order to sustain competitive advantage.

Purpose of the Book

This book provides a practical strategic approach to initiating and implementing innovation within healthcare organizations. It defines the factors that enable innovation success in healthcare, with reference to all stages of innovation and with a particular focus on the role of clinical and organizational leadership in effecting innovation.

Who is the Book For

The book is aimed not only at doctor leaders and other clinical innovators, researchers and strategists working across the public and private healthcare sectors, but also healthcare executives, healthcare system leaders and commissioners. I hope that it will provide the readers with practical guidance on applying leadership effectively at different innovation stages, in order for innovations to succeed and be sustained long-term. Through the lens of real-life organizations and real-life innovation processes,

For Michael, Paul, Angelina and Panos

I am describing the interaction between innovation stakeholders, the challenges that innovators face, how leadership works or doesn't work and in what circumstances, as well as the influence of internal and external stakeholders in the success and failure of innovations.

About This Book

I am very proud to publish this piece of work as a result of my passion for innovation and leadership in healthcare. This book is about sharing the experiences of contemporary healthcare organizations that have gone through their journeys of innovation and transformation and have learned through their successes and failures. This book is destined to inform, educate and inspire healthcare leaders, who are looking to balance innovation, transformation and risk in the current volatile and ambiguous environment.

I am extremely privileged to have lived and breathed two different healthcare organizations during their innovation and transformation change over a period of four years and have learned from their successes and failures. The experiences I have gained as a healthcare leader facilitating, enacting, effecting and observing innovation processes and outcomes are of huge value, which I have managed to capture and describe in this book.

The COVID-19 pandemic has been a challenging time for the healthcare sector and the healthcare system changes that so far have followed the pandemic have been disruptive. This book has captured the pre- and post-pandemic state of innovation, including the creation of the integrated care systems which have influenced the innovation mindset of healthcare providers.

For that reason, I feel this manual is probably the most contemporary piece of qualitative research on innovation and leadership within healthcare organizations.

Coventry, UK   Dr Penny Kechagioglou

Contents

1 **Why Publish About Healthcare Innovation and What is the Problem We Are Trying to Solve**   1
   1.1 Defining Innovation   2
   1.2 Defining Leadership   3
   1.3 A Surge of Innovation   5
   1.4 The Problem   6
   1.5 The Focus on Leadership   7
   References   8

2 **What We Know from Existing Theories of Innovation**   11
   2.1 Innovation Theories   11
   2.2 Leadership Theories   22
   2.3 Enablers and Barriers to Innovation Success   26
   2.4 Resistance to Change   32
   References   35

3 Learning from Innovation Failure—*A Case Study* — 41
- 3.1 Idea Generation — 42
- 3.2 The Ideas Den — 47
- 3.3 The Innovation Team — 49
- 3.4 Stakeholder Engagement and The Evaluation Process — 55
- 3.5 The Final Decision About Innovation Adoption — 61
- 3.6 Lessons on Leadership — 64
- 3.7 Why Did the Innovation Fail — 72
- 3.8 Organizational Response to Innovation Failure — 77
- References — 79

4 Learning from Innovation Success—*A Case Study* — 83
- 4.1 The Innovation Purpose — 84
- 4.2 Leadership Enablers and Barriers to Innovation — 91
- 4.3 Perception of the Innovation Process and Leadership by Stakeholders — 105
- 4.4 Deep Dive into Leadership at Different Innovation Stages — 110
- 4.5 Balancing Innovation, Transformation and Risk — 122
- 4.6 Why Did the Innovation Program Succeed — 123
- References — 128

5 Using Learnings to Make a Model of Innovation Success — 131
- 5.1 The Preliminary Model of Innovation — 131
- References — 142

6 Model Validation in Real-Time—*A Case Study* — 143
6.1 Application of the New Model in a New Context — 144
6.2 Lessons Learned from a Complex Leadership and Innovation Context — 155
References — 164

7 A Contemporary Framework of Leadership in Innovation — 165
7.1 Leadership Lessons for Innovation Success — 165
7.2 Final Model for Leadership in Innovation Success — 169

Appendix A: Methodology — 171

Epilogue — 175

1

Why Publish About Healthcare Innovation and What is the Problem We Are Trying to Solve

Abstract Global healthcare systems are facing challenging times in an effort to sustain financially and reputationally in a continually changing, volatile and unpredictable environment. The adoption, implementation and spread of innovation in complex healthcare organizations is considered the prerequisite for success, bridging patient care, funding and wellbeing gaps (Bessant and Davis 1999). Innovation has always been at the top of the National Health Service (NHS) sustainability agenda (Dixon-Woods et al. 2011; NHS Confederation 2021; NHS England 2019) but more so recently and following the global pandemic in 2020. The private healthcare sector has traditionally paved the way to innovation and entrepreneurship with its commercial business nature, but even the private sector has been challenged during the recent pandemic. Both the UK NHS and the private healthcare sectors are currently undergoing an intense period of service recovery as well as service transformation which is characterized by innovation acceleration. This book on healthcare innovation success comes at the right time when global healthcare systems are striving to return to their pre-pandemic operational state, whilst at the same time designing and implementing innovative services.

1.1 Defining Innovation

The definition of innovation may differ between organizations, depending on the individual organizational methods of innovation. However, the principles that define innovation are similar and can be summarized as 'the activities of an organization that help improve its performance' (Rogers 1998). Those activities may include the development of new products or services, the improvement of existing products or services, knowledge creation, training program development, the creation of new technology or intellectual property (Rogers 1998). Innovation in healthcare involves the process of idea creation, diffusion and implementation which could be a linear or a cyclical process, sometimes described as a 'messy' process due to stakeholder complexities. Innovation adoption and diffusion (spread) is influenced by several enablers and barriers, which may differ depending on the organizational context. It is the balance of enablers and barriers which sometimes leads to a differential adoption and diffusion of innovation within complex healthcare organizations, even in the same healthcare environment.

Healthcare innovation is often initiated by clinical leaders on the front line who are the subject matter experts and who can suggest and drive solutions to common and emerging healthcare problems. Innovation is also often driven by leaders higher up in the organizational hierarchy, organizations. The NHS has traditionally been considered an internal-facing organizations with little or no employee control over innovation ideation and implementation. The introduction of Integrated Care Systems in April 2021 has already started to challenge the current status quo of the NHS with the development of a new national strategy for innovation (NHS Confederation 2021). The implementation of the national innovation strategy should bring the NHS closer to its private and voluntary sector partners, who have enriched their innovation processes and capabilities in order to sustain themselves financially.

1.3 A Surge of Innovation

The NHS Integrated Care System reform has come at the same time as the NHS is recovering and restoring services after the COVID-19 pandemic. The pandemic has resulted in a healthcare crisis, rapid change and innovation disruption. The NHS is now in the unique position of having the knowledge of innovation successes and failures during the global pandemic to be able to drive the healthcare innovation agenda. Healthcare leaders have experienced examples of effective as well as ineffective system leadership to draw upon in leading on the national healthcare innovation agenda (Currie et al. 2021). Harnessing the leadership knowledge and skills acquired during the pandemic, working across systems, will enable the NHS to innovate faster and safer. The international standards organization has published the new innovation management standard in 2019 which states (Brady 2020): 'An organization can innovate more effectively and efficiently if all necessary activities and other interrelated or interacting elements are managed as a system'.

1.4 The Problem

Although healthcare leaders are aware of the need to change their business strategy and innovate more, there is ambiguity as to what practical steps they could take to optimize innovation adoption, diffusion and implementation success. Innovation benefits and their translation into clear deliverables is a challenge for healthcare leaders and also how to achieve sustainable innovation.

Innovation diffusion requires unique organizational leadership capabilities and considerable organizational change capability (Greenhalgh and Papoutsi 2019), which is why healthcare lacks behind other industries when it comes to innovation (Bates et al. 2017). Despite attempts by some NHS organizations to promote innovation through multiple stakeholder engagement (open innovation), there is often lack of an organized implementation strategy for innovation in the NHS. Innovative ideas may not become diffused beyond local adoption and innovation champions who are usually front-line clinicians often become disillusioned as a result.

The commonest triggers for disruptive innovation in healthcare include competition from new market entries, technological developments and changes in political, legal and social rules, all potentially leading to new customer demands (Bessant and Tidd 2013). To be able to respond to those triggers, healthcare organizations need to be in a state of 'innovation alertness' driven by internal inspirational leaders, who manage the innovation agenda effectively. In addition, healthcare organizations need to proactively build their innovation infrastructure and capabilities in order to respond to external contextual triggers (exploration). At the same time, they need to be able to continue with their business-as-usual activities (exploitation) whilst innovating, avoiding conflict between those two processes. The leadership styles required to balance exploration and exploitation activities within organizations may vary and they are key to innovation success (Oke et al. 2008).

Few healthcare organizations have continued to innovate disruptively as a means of differentiation and competitive advantage. Those that have managed to do so are often driven by leaders who exhibit unique entrepreneurial characteristics such as agility, bravery, autonomy, risk-taking behaviours and they have established robust reward and incentivization systems for their staff (Bessant and Tidd 2013; Kuratko et al. 2014). The term 'entrepreneurship' is closely related to 'innovation' and in the context of existing organizations, entrepreneurship can be defined as the start of new and innovative ventures (Gartner 1990).

1.5 The Focus on Leadership

Healthcare organizations operate in a dynamic and competitive environment which requires them to balance disruptive innovation and sustainable implementation (Boer and Gertsen 2003). Clinical and organizational leadership has been identified as one of the most important enablers for innovation success in the NHS (Jones et al. 2019; Koryak et al. 2018) but the role of leadership at different stages of the innovation process needs to be better defined. Clinical and non-clinical leaders in both the public and private healthcare sectors would benefit from a clear guide to optimizing innovation adoption, diffusion and implementation.

This book aims to consolidate knowledge around leadership behaviours and leadership approaches and their role in making innovation adoption, diffusion and implementation a success within complex healthcare organizations. It will attempt to do that through the study and analysis of three real-life innovation cases in the public and private healthcare sectors.

References

Bass BM (1988) The inspirational processes of leadership. J Manag Dev 7:21–31

Bates DW, Sheikh A, Asch DA (2017) Innovative environments in healthcare: where and how new approaches to care are succeeding. Health Affairs 36(3)

Bessant J, Davis F (1999) Developing strategic continuous improvement capability. Int J Oper Prod Manag 19(11):1106–1119

Bessant J, Tidd J (2013) Managing innovation, 5th edn. Wiley. ISBN: 978-1-118-53859-3

Boer H, Gertsen F (2003). From continuous improvement to continuous innovation: a (retro)(per)spective. Int J Technol Manag 26(8)

Brady A (2020) The virtuous circe of innovation management. ISOFocus

Currie G, Gulati K, Sohal A et al (2021) Distributing systems level leadership to address the COVID-19 pandemic. BMJ Leader 0:1–6. https://doi.org/10.1136/leader-2020-000280

Dixon-Woods M, Amalberti R, Goodman S et al (2011) Problems and promises of innovation: why healthcare needs to rethink its love/hate relationship with the new. BMJ Qual Safety 20(suppl 1):i45–i51

Frieden TR (2014) Six components necessary for effective public health program implementation. Am J Public Health 104:17–22

Gartner WB (1990) What are we talking about when we talk about entrepreneurship? J Bus Ventur 5:15–28

Greenhalgh T, Papoutsi C (2019) Spreading and scaling up innovation and improvement. BMJ 365:I2068

Jones B, Horton T, Walburton W (2019) The improvement journey. The Health Foundation

Koryak O, Lockett A, Hayton J et al (2018) Disentangling the antecedents of ambidexterity: exploration and exploitation. Res Policy 47(2018):413–427

Kuratko DF, Hornsby JS, Covin JG (2014) Diagnosing a firm's internal environment for corporate entrepreneurship. Bus Horiz 57:37–47

NHS England (2019) Breaking down barriers to better healthcare

NHS Confederation (2021) Integration and innovation: working together to improve health and social care for all

Oke A, Munshi N, Walumbwa MO (2008) The Influence of Leadership on Innovation Processes and Activities. Organ Dyn 38(1):64–72

Rogers EM (1998) The definition and measurement of innovation. The Melbourne Institute working paper No. 10/98

Rostain M (2021) The impact of organizational culture on entrepreneurial orientation: a meta-analysis. J Bus Ventur Insights 15:e00234

Silva A (2016) What is leadership?. J Bus Stud Q 8(1)

Waldman DA, Bass BM (1991) Transformational leadership at different phases of the innovation process. J High Technol Manag Res 2(2):169–180

2

What We Know from Existing Theories of Innovation

Abstract Dissemination of lessons learned from innovative activities in terms of what has worked well and what has not work as well, is a characteristic of learning organizations where innovation is at the top of their strategic agenda. Healthcare organizations often struggle integrating training on continuous improvement into their systems. As a result, they often fail to evaluate the implementation of innovation and share lessons learned. This results in innovations often failing to diffuse and scale following local adoption. This section gives a summary of the most pertinent theories on innovation and leadership relevant to healthcare.

2.1 Innovation Theories

Healthcare innovations are new ideas, processes or services aiming at improving performance such as achieving better healthcare quality, safety, clinical outcomes as well as reducing healthcare costs (Social Care Institute for Excellence 2018). The process of innovation involves the communication and application of innovation within a population or system. Innovation processes aim at implementing new ideas or processes within organisations or systems, which in turn can benefit the organisation, population or system (Omachonu and Einspruch 2010; Albury 2005).

The process of innovation usually begins with idea creation, followed by idea adoption and resulting in the innovation being implemented (West 2002; Fleuren and Wiefferink 2004), leading to innovation commitment (Greenhalgh et al. 2004). The Innovation Diffusion theory was introduced in 1962 by Rogers, was developed further in 1995 and the theory focuses on the rate of spread of innovations including technological innovations amongst populations (Wani and Ali 2015). Innovation diffusion is a social process that involves multiple stakeholders.

The traditional *Diffusion of Innovation theory (DOI)* created by Rogers, consists of five stages in a linear fashion (Wani and Ali 2015; Martins et al. 2016) as described below; the focus of this theory is on the innovation itself rather than the context of innovation:

1. Knowledge creation about the innovation;
2. Persuasion to adopt the innovation;
3. Decision-making to adopt the innovation;
4. Innovation implementation and
5. Confirmation or reinforcement of the innovation.

Out of those five stages, there are usually three stages that are most commonly used, as follows: *idea creation* (corresponding to stages 1 and 2 above), *adoption* (corresponding to stage 3) and *implementation* (corresponding to stages 4 and 5).

According to Rogers (1995), successfully adopted innovations are the ones which bring a relative advantage over conventional practice, they are compatible with the wider organizational context and culture, have low complexity, can be trialed and have an observable impact.

Contextual conditions of the healthcare system where innovation takes place play some enabling role in the adoption and diffusion of innovation. For example, any prior innovation knowledge and experience, the degree of innovativeness in the system culture, the perceived need for innovation by the users and the adequacy of communication channels, are all important enablers for the successful adoption and diffusion of innovation (Wani and Ali 2015; Rogers 1995). In the case of technological innovations, human factors and the organizational context play a key role in their adoption. The human factor element may involve customer engagement, training on the use and the monitoring of new technologies (Batt-Rawden et al. 2017).

There are two other innovation diffusion theories which are particular pertinent in the adoption and diffusion of technological innovation and consider the organizational context as well as the external environment to a greater degree than the Diffusion of Innovation theory; these are the TOE and the INT theories (Martins et al. 2016; Yang et al. 2015; Chen et al. 2021):

1. The *Technology—Organization—Environment (TOE) theory* of technological innovation diffusion considers the importance of the organizational culture and readiness for innovation internally in the organization and externally in the whole system—market forces, economy, social context, health inequalities. This theory focuses mainly on the organizational context as an innovation enabler (knowledge, training, expertise,

leadership and management support, organizational size and business needs).
2. The *Institutional Theory of Innovation (INT) diffusion* supports that the internal organizational innovation decisions are influenced by the environment where the organization operates. This theory focuses mainly on environmental factors as innovation enablers (competitor and partner pressure, government support, socio-economical and technological factors).

Innovation adoption is a prerequisite to innovation diffusion. Innovation adoption makes the innovation idea legitimate at a small scale and innovation diffusion involves the spread of innovation through the population (Barlow 2013). Innovation diffusion relies on effective marketing and communication channels which enable innovation to spread within organizations and populations (Sahin 2006). Innovation diffusion refers to the passive spread of innovation or the 'active' innovation dissemination which involves the activity of persuading others to adopt innovation (Greenhalgh et al. 2004).

The diffusion of innovations is influenced by the behaviour of adopters, which is in turn is influenced by interpersonal contacts and social interaction within and between communities (Valente and Davis 1995). The implementation phase of innovation is complex, critical for innovation diffusion success and often requires considerable organization change (Counte and Meurer 2001).

According to Rogers (1995), there are five categories of innovation adopters—*the Innovators, the Early Adopters, the Early Majority, the Late Majority and the Laggards.*

There are certain leadership characteristics that early innovation adopters should possess in order to positively influence innovation adoption within healthcare organizations; those include (West 2002; Greenhalgh et al. 2004; Waldman and Bass 1991):

- A shared vision with the rest of the organization;
- The ability to influence and motivate people to challenge the status quo;
- The ability to work collaboratively with various stakeholders towards the shared vision, whilst navigating resistance to change.

The above unique characteristics of early adopters—*shared vision, influence and impact, collaboration*, differentiates early adopters from the early majority and makes them more likely to succeed in moving innovation from the adoption to the diffusion phase (Wani and Ali 2015).

The role of key opinion leaders and innovation champions in engaging and motivating stakeholders during the innovation diffusion phase is key; they are usually but not always the earliest adopters themselves. Their role in endorsing new ideas and influencing behaviour change is a catalyst to the success of innovation diffusion (Valente and Pumpuang 2007). It is often the creation of a critical mass of supporters and advocates of the innovation that is required for innovation diffusion success (Ash 1997).

Different leadership skills are required at different stages of the innovation process, ranging from creativity and transformational skills at the ideation phase (exploration), to coordination and transactional skills at the implementation (exploitation) and diffusion phase (Oke et al. 2008). The balance of exploration and exploitation in the case of innovation is likely to give healthcare organizations competitive advantage, by ensuring that great ideas are implemented safely and sustainably. Patients and customers are looking for excellence in service quality and organizations have to balance the high investment risk of disruptive innovation with the continuous quality improvement element of innovation. Fast-growing healthcare organizations often need to invest in disruptive innovation to gain competitive advantage (Oke et al. 2008), but this investment should not conflict with the clinical governance and quality aspects of care which features in continuous innovation processes.

Omachonu and Einspruch (2010) proposed that innovation can be a *complex and 'messy' process*, with a range of different stakeholders and stakeholder partnerships involved during innovation diffusion. Unlike Rogers' linear model, Omachonu' model supports the collaboration between partners in the innovation diffusion phase of the process, including clinicians and care givers, patients and consumer advocacy groups, innovator companies, universities and regulatory agencies (Omachonu and Einspruch 2010). The non-linear nature of the model offers to innovators the flexibility to start innovation work at different phases in the process and through various channels. Innovation success in such a complex model depends largely on a transformational leadership style of the healthcare leaders involved, which encourages a positive approach to change and creates a safe learning environment for innovation to thrive. On the other hand, a transactional leadership style is more suited in the case of innovation implementation, which needs structuring and policy development, as well as in the evaluation of innovation implementation (Waldman and Bass 1991; Oke et al. 2008). Incorporating an evaluation of innovation implementation into the process of innovation could support with validating the innovation, legitimising it and allowing the dissemination of innovation outcomes which can maximise innovation diffusion (Sahin 2006).

Berwick (2003) suggested that healthcare innovation ideation in much easier than innovation implementation and diffusion, because the latter two stages involve some degree of organizational change. He highlighted the role of clinical and organizational leadership as an important enabler in innovation change; clinical leaders should influence stakeholder perception of innovation and ensure they are aligned with organisational vision. Clinical leaders are just as important as their followers who could act as innovation champions, supporting and propagating their leader message about the role of innovation, increasing the chances of innovation diffusion.

The power of the early adopters of innovation is also as strong as the power of non-adopters who exhibit resistance to change. The presence of effective clinical leadership which collaborates well with the management team can be critical in converting non-adopters to innovation supporters. There are other factors that determine the success of innovation diffusion within healthcare organizations, which also rely on strong leadership capabilities. Those include: the development of scientifically and technologically sound innovative ideas, the presence of strong product management skills in the organization and the presence of an active marketing team who is fully aligned with the innovation vision and strategy (Berwick 2003).

de Ven (2017) described a *Cyclical Innovation Model* unlike Rogers (1995) and Omachonu and Einspruch (2010). He described the dynamic interaction between innovation creation and innovation implementation, in the form of divergent behaviours (creation) and convergent behaviours (execution). Those behaviours exist interchangeably and shape the final status of innovation. Several enabling and constraining factors prevail during this process, interacting in a dynamic manner and influencing the outcome of innovations. The outcome is unpredictable but can be steered by organisational leadership (de Ven 2017).

The implementation phase of the innovation process is the period between the decision to adopt the innovation and the routine and consistent use within the organization by the majority of its stakeholders, which is a period of intense skillset and knowledge building (Klein and Sorra 1996; Damschroder et al. 2009). Strategic implementation of innovations is crucial to every business success and if badly executed, can have a catastrophic effect to the business bottom line and reputation (Pryor et al. 2007). The implementation stage in the innovation process can be seen as a catalyst stage, because it determines whether the innovation becomes routine practice or is dismissed (Fleuren and Wiefferink 2004). In addition, implementation is an active and social process, involving the interaction between individuals and organizations, the inner context (culture, structure, politics) and the outer context (social, political, economical). The interaction between the inner and the outer context is important in understanding and resolving barriers to innovation implementation (Damschroder et al. 2009; May et al. 2016).

The implementation phase often comes later in the innovation process and is often seen as separate to strategic thinking within organizations. Van Limburg et al. (2011) claims that innovation implementation should begin earlier in the innovation process and be considered at the strategic stage, when there is intense brainstorming, knowledge creation and persuasion (Limburg et al. 2011). Technological innovations in healthcare are likely to influence a wider sociotechnical network (Greenhalgh et al. 2012; Mikhailova 2018) and their implementation should begin early into the strategic phase (May et al. 2016). By doing so, potential implementation threats can be addressed early such as resistance to adoption from clinicians and other key stakeholders.

Several authors have suggested the following enablers for the successful implementation of innovation within healthcare organizations (Greenhalgh et al. 2004; Ross et al. 2016):

- Supportive organizational structures;
- Visionary top leadership;
- Competent workforce;
- Ongoing funding sources;
- Key stakeholder communication and alignment with culture and values.

Bourgeois and Brodwin (1984) proposed the *Cultural Strategic Model* to show that innovation implementation can be embedded within organizational cultures when staff at all levels are involved in the innovation design and implementation process. He concludes that when strategic implementation is part of the organizational culture, the effort spent implementing the strategy is much less (Bourgeois and Brodwin 1984).

Van Limburg et al. (2011) refers to *Business Modelling* as an effective innovation implementation strategy, enabling the evaluation of innovation at the early stages of the innovation process. Business modelling allows broad stakeholder involvement earlier in the innovation process, co-creation of solutions with key stakeholders and earlier problem-solving, which has positive influence on innovation diffusion success (Van Limburg et al. 2011; Gemert-Pijnen et al. 2011).

Successful innovation implementation does not guarantee sustainable innovation diffusion (Klein and Sorra 1996). Global healthcare systems are in need of sustainable innovations, those that remain beyond the trial phase. To maximise innovation diffusion and sustainability in the healthcare sector and in different global systems, there are different factors that need to be considered to those that facilitate early adoption (Martin and Waring 2012). These are:

- The presence of supportive networks within and between organizations;
- The existence of active innovation champions;
- Robust mechanisms for innovation evaluation;
- Mechanisms for monitoring and responding to user feedback.

The recruitment of an entrepreneurial workforce, who possess the clinical and technological expertise as well as the creative and leadership abilities would add significantly to the innovation capabilities of any healthcare organization (Hunter et al. 2012).

Scaling healthcare innovations beyond a single system and in a sustainable fashion, often requires the set up and evaluation of innovation in a small scalable unit before moving into full scale. This process involves considerable amount of experimentation, robust data collection and analysis, strong organizational leadership and open stakeholder communication (Barker et al. 2016). Learning from other healthcare organisations who succeeded in implementing innovations is critical. Shared learnings can be achieved through publications, blogs, webinars, conferences and other forms of networking.

Crompton-Phillips (2020) describes a model of innovation diffusion which aligns well with Greenhalgh et al. (2004) implementation theory and May et al. (2016) whole system approach to change theory: the essential model components include the creation of a Vision to solve a wicked problem *(the 'Why')*, the inclusion and trust on key opinion leaders *(the 'Who')*, the continuous collection, display and analysis of Data *(the 'What')*, the use of data to guide Capacity building (*the 'How'*) and the creation of Alignment between incentivisation and sustainable behavioural change (*the 'What's in It for me'*). The same author described examples of US organisations who adopted the framework and have seen various innovations being spread and sustained. The learnings from this model include the importance of a shared organizational vision and strong transformational leadership in influencing stakeholder engagement in innovation. The transformational leadership style needs to be balanced with a transactional leadership style, which will ensure a reward and incentivisation system for achieving innovation goals.

The application of innovation diffusion models in healthcare organizations requires a supportive organizational environment, described as *Organizational Resilience*. Fukofuka and Lokke (2015) refers to organizational resilience as a combination of employee and organizational qualities which create a robust and resourceful environment during periods of uncertainty or crisis. When those qualities are expanded further to include aspects of organizational behavior such as trust, employee autonomy and authentic leadership, there seems to be a positive correlation between those qualities and organizational resilience (Fukofuka and Lokke 2015). Resilience engineering refers to the organizational attitude to change and incorporates strategies that prevent system failures and resistance, which can be applied to innovation processes as well (Nemeth et al. 2008). The strategies suggested for prevention of system resistance and failure are dependent on team working, challenge recognition, resource reallocation, collective response to change and learning from errors (Nemeth et al. 2008). Innovation processes within healthcare organizations involve considerable change and the risk of failure is high which makes the theory of resilience engineering very relevant. Organizational leadership supporting a resilient culture of innovation is likely to have a positive effect towards innovation diffusion success.

2.2 Leadership Theories

Leadership in the context of complex organizations is defined by Yukl (2006) within Weintraub and McKee (2019), as an influencing and facilitating process for achieving shared objectives. In terms of individual leadership traits and their link to innovation diffusion, there is evidence to suggest that transformational leadership within healthcare organizations plays a key role throughout the five stages of the diffusion of innovation process, but particularly in the early stages of ideation and the intention to adopt (Martins et al. 2016; Carreiro and Oliveira 2019). The aspects of transformational leadership that are particularly helpful in driving the adoption and diffusion of innovation include the following (Carreiro and Oliveira 2019):

1. *Articulation and communication of a shared vision* for innovation by senior managers and leaders—the 'Why', also described in Crompton-Phillips (2020);
2. *The intellectual stimulation of followers* around innovation by leaders and senior managers—the 'How' can we do things differently;
3. *Follower incentivisation and support* from senior managers and leaders that drives internal motivation and investment on the common vision from the followers—the 'What's in it for me'.

Organizational behaviour plays a critical role in the behaviour of individual leaders and followers as well as the attitude of teams towards innovation. Aspects of Organizational behaviour that determine the success of innovation, include structures and hierarchies (power dynamics), experts (champions, training, human resources), supportive leadership, communication and a culture of experimentation (Ash and Lorenzi 2017).

The *Crescive Strategic model* has been proposed by Bourgeois and Brodwin (1984) and gives power to middle managers within organizations to become strategic champions, ensuring that strategy implementation begins as early as strategy formulation. The other important lesson from Bourgeois' model is that middle managers are best placed to facilitate communication channels between top managers and front-line people within organizations, with the aim of effecting innovation success. When it comes to innovation implementation, developing and preserving a culture of openness and transparency amongst organizational stakeholders may facilitate strategic implementation (Birken et al. 2011).

Front line staff work at the core of every business and are best placed to drive strategic innovation. *Distributed* leadership in the context of innovation, moves power from top down to bottom up and can lead to a more effective and faster innovation adoption, with less risk of employee resistance as well as more sustainable benefits (Martin and Waring 2012). Although top managers may have little technical knowledge compared to front line leaders, they have the available resources to make innovations happen. Front line leaders are technical experts but without resources to make innovations happen, which could lead to innovations stalling at an early stage without any top manager (executive) support (McKee et al. 2013). A collaboration between top managers and front-line leaders has been suggested as a potential model for innovation success (McKee et al. 2013) for the reason that the combination of skills, knowledge and power from the collaboration is more likely to lead to the desired innovation outcomes. Helfrich et al. (2007) also advocates that innovation implementation should be an organizational rather than an individual priority in complex healthcare organizations.

This combined top-down and bottom-up leadership model has also been represented as the *Tight-Loose-Tight model* (Crompton-Phillips 2020). The latter model supports a bottom-up approach to innovation strategy and a top-down influence for creating the vision and promoting a system-wide approach to change. This alignment between top managers and front-line leaders can mitigate against any cultural differences between those two groups which can hinder innovation outcomes. This cultural conflict is particularly prevalent in healthcare and occurs because clinical staff focus mainly on individual patient outcomes and top managers focus mainly on organisational benefits (Mannion and Davies 2018). Cultural alignment amongst healthcare teams, respecting each other's innovation goals, responding to triggers in a synergistic way and sharing common values, increases the chance of innovation diffusion (Mannion and Davies 2018).

The *Triple Helix innovation model* was developed in the 1990s (Etzkowitz 2013; Ranga and Etzkowitz 2013) and describes the unique partnership between government organizations, academia and industry in an effort to accelerate innovation diffusion. The helix is characterised by its triad components (state, industry and academia) working together in partnership and with the aim of achieving knowledge transfer, whilst managing key interdependencies (Ranga and Etzkowitz 2013). The concept is very similar to Omachonu's innovation model (Omachonu and Einspruch 2010), which incorporates partnerships between public organizations, industry and academia to develop and accelerate innovations. According to Etzkowitz (2013), the interactions between different institutional spheres promotes a self-sustaining innovation culture and a state of innovation synergy. The application of the triple helix innovation model in healthcare results in the combination of resources, skills and knowledge which facilitates the implementation and diffusion of innovations. Innovation can be seen as a form of co-creation between the innovators (healthcare organizations), the developers of the technology (industry, university) and the customers (Nilsen et al. 2016). Interorganisational partnerships are considered to be a prerequisite to successful dissemination of innovations and can be catalysts for innovation diffusion and sustainability (Barnett et al. 2011).

Collaboration and shared leadership are the two dimensions of the *Distributed Leadership model*, both being enabling factors for innovation diffusion in healthcare organizations (Currie and Spyridonidis 2018). The actors involved in this leadership model are usually top managers who lead on resources and culture, doctors who lead on resource allocation, commissioning and peer motivation and nurses who lead on front line staff motivation and awareness. This innovation model escapes from the traditional top-down hierarchical healthcare model: a senior manager or executive initiates the innovation strategic direction which is then driven by front line subject matter experts (nurses/doctors), but there is shared leadership amongst the three parties (executives/doctors/nurses). Shared leadership between executives and front-line clinical leaders becomes more prominent with time. Doctors play the facilitator role for innovation delivery as well as the essential link between front line staff and top managers (Currie and Spyridonidis 2018).

Distributed leadership is a characteristic of the *Open Innovation model*, defined as the inflows of knowledge from external networks into the organization and the outflow of knowledge from the organization to external stakeholders. The purpose of open innovation is the acceleration of innovation processes and capabilities as well as the diffusion of innovations to other markets (Chesbrough and Bogers 2014). In healthcare systems, open innovation allows the boundaries between public and private organizations to be lifted. Ideas and knowledge transfer become easier amongst innovators, leaders and followers and internal and external capabilities join up to maximise innovation diffusion (Chesbrough and Bogers 2014).

The *Cyclical Innovation model* (Berkhout et al. 2006) recognises that innovation is not a linear process, it can be triggered at any point and is so influential that one successful innovation can drive more innovation. This model is applicable to young and entrepreneurial organizations which aim at creating multiple differentiators which if put together, can create a unique service proposition for customers. This is a social innovation model which is characterised by a strong sense of organizational vision, a risky organizational behaviour, and one that values partnerships within and between organizations (Bessant and Tidd 2013).

2.3 Enablers and Barriers to Innovation Success

Some barriers to successful innovation diffusion include the presence of professional silos, the lack of available clinical and managerial time and the lack of innovation funds (Cresswell et al. 2016). According to Greenhalgh et al. (2017), there is also the lack of effective networking and information sharing within and between teams that disables innovation implementation and diffusion. Greenhalgh et al. (2018) and her team have developed and published the NASSS technological innovation model, which refers to the non-adoption, abandonment, spread, scale-up and sustainability model, addressing enablers and barriers to technological innovation diffusion. The NASSS model has been applied to six technology-enabled programs and explained why some innovations succeed in being diffused and others fail (Greenhalgh et al. 2017, 2018). The components of the model co-exist interdependently and include:

- the clinical unmet need addressed by the innovation;
- the value-added effect of the innovation;
- the perceived ease of use;
- the degree of organizational readiness for implementation;
- the characteristics of early adopters and champions of innovation;
- the degree of organizational resilience to change and
- the effects of the socio-political context in innovation adoption and diffusion.

Borins (2002) in Micheli et al. (2015) described three barriers to adoption of technological innovation in the public sector and those include:

- resistance to change due to conflicting stakeholder priorities;
- risk aversion towards innovation failure and
- strict hierarchical structures.

Van Limburg et al. (2011) emphasized the importance of stakeholder interaction in the development and implementation of healthcare technologies. One particular stakeholder who is often neglected in the early stages of innovation is the patient and public community. Patients are often the end users of healthcare innovations and they have the power to advocate for and against innovations, enabling those which can have the highest value and impact to them.

Llewellyn et al. (2014) described the wider socio-political issues faced by the public healthcare sector that may hinder technological innovation diffusion, even when there is clinical evidence of benefit. Such factors can lead to poor innovation implementation, through reducing the chances of innovations being funded, creating misalignment between clinicians and managers and resulting in further innovation stifling. The factors include:

– organizational power relationships;
– the political stance of top managers;
– innovation reimbursement issues and
– non-innovator resistance.

Some authors support the presence of quantitative evidence of innovation benefit as an enabler for innovation adoption and diffusion (Barnett et al. 2011; Ferlie et al. 2005). Barnett et al. (2011) explored the views of clinicians and found that the presence of quantitative evidence could make innovations more likely to diffuse. There is a risk of early over-adoption of an innovation without enough evidence, which can make stakeholders lose trust on the innovation and leaders may lose their credibility. The role of inner organizational and inter-organizational relationships is key in making sense of the available evidence leading most likely to innovation adoption rather than abandonment (Ferlie et al. 2005).

Table 2.1 Enablers, barriers and opportunities for Innovation diffusion

Enablers	Barriers	Opportunities	Author(s)
Cross sectional collaborations	Service based tariffs Low per capita spending Privacy & security directives Clinician time for innovation Low risk-taking behaviour	Move to value-based innovation Launching national innovation centres	Cresswell et al. (2016)
Organisational capabilities, behaviour and culture	Low patient motivation Lack of champions Low clinician acceptance Interoperability issues Inadequate IT support/staff Data protection concerns Inadequate policy/implementation strategy No plausible business case		Greenhalgh et al. (2017)
Stakeholder participation Co-creation	Poor evaluation of innovation impact	Business modelling Persuasive tech design Human-centred design	van Gemert-Pijnen et al. (2011)
Stakeholder participation Co-creation	Financial structures Legislations lagging behind Reluctance to use Poor scalability Complex interdependencies		van Limburg et al. (2011)

(continued)

Table 2.1 (continued)

Enablers	Barriers	Opportunities	Author(s)
Block grants for innovation	NHS architecture (silos)	Learning collaboratives	Collins (2018)
Learn from other industries		Innovation hubs	
Early physician involvement			Blumenthal and Kilo (1998)
Emphasizing patient benefits			
Investment in IT			
Board support			
Educate teams to change	Discontinued funds/stalled pilots		Verna et al. (2013)
Evaluate health outcomes	No cross-border collaboration		
Economic analysis	Knowledge not shared/power politics		
	Unwillingness to scale up		
	Large datasets and MDTs		Cresswell et al. (2016)
	Poor evaluation of impact		
Clinician engagement/ training			Mair et al. (2012)
Local champions			
Funding and policies			
Patient experience			

(continued)

Table 2.1 (continued)

Enablers	Barriers	Opportunities	Author(s)
Clinician engagement Competent IT project team Potential for development System usable/ little training needed	No time in job plan for implementation Unstable internal environment, high cost		Ovretvbt et al. (2007)
Stakeholder alignment Scientific evidence Training		Learning from other centre experience	Denis et al. (2002)
	Lack of vision, low risk taking History of poor implementation No middle manager support		Conner (2004)
	No funding/ available time/internal incentives		Bloch and Bugge (2013)
	Short-term budgets and planning horizons Poor skills in risk and change management Few rewards or incentives, admin burden, cultural constraints, risk aversion		Albury (2005)

The summary of published key enablers to innovation diffusion success are as follows (Table 2.1):

- organizational leadership and culture;
- stakeholder engagement and cross system collaborations;
- concurrent strategic innovation ideation, implementation and evaluation;
- organizational vision and innovation champions;
- funding streams and internal organization capabilities.

The summary of published key barriers to innovation diffusion success are as follows (Table 2.1):

- lack of clinician incentivisation;
- resistance to change and lack of effective change management process;
- lack of scientific evidence;
- organizational risk aversion;
- lack of middle management support.

2.4 Resistance to Change

Resistance to innovation is defined as a reaction to new products and services which brings about a change or upsets the status quo. The degree of resistance depends on how threatening the change is perceived by consumers (Mani and Chouk 2018). Ram and Sheth's model (1989) and Mani and Chouk (2018) explain resistance to service innovation by consumers in terms of five barriers:

- innovation is perceived as complex to use and/or highly priced (perceived value);
- innovation is perceived as a security risk;

- there is image incongruence with the organization or system;
- there is perceived lack of human interaction.

Mani and Chouk (2018) added three more barriers to the model, including technological vulnerability and overdependency, skepticism about new technology and individual resistance to change in status quo. Braithwaite (2018) addresses resistance to change in healthcare from a systems leadership perspective, including the presence of bureaucracy, a top-down decision-making process, a blocking political culture and a lack of clinical leadership to influence change.

Judson (1999) saw resistance to change as a continuous process leading eventually to commitment to change. Coetsee (1999) described resistance to change as progression from aggressive (high resistance) to passive (low resistance) before reaching commitment. The model of resistance—acceptance differs from Ram and Sheth's model of innovation resistance, the latter focusing only on barriers to innovation with no eventual commitment.

Herscovitch and Meyer (2002) subsequently described commitment as a continuum from compliance to cooperation and finally championing, the latter being one of the most important enablers in implementing and spreading innovation. Coetsee's latest theory (2011), states that people are initially apathetic when it comes to change and they move down a resistance or commitment path according to their impressions of the contextual situation.

The downside of the above models of resistance to change when applied to innovation, is that they are looking at the individual level, ignoring the group, organization and system level. Lewin's research around group dynamics demonstrated the positive impact of group behaviours in the change process, through engagement, communication, motivation and conflict resolution (Burnes 2014).

Lapointe and Rivard (2005) later supported the theory that individual behaviours need to be considered together with group behaviours (system resistance) and that resistance to change needs to be managed early in the innovation process. They identified five interdependent components of resistance, including:

- individual resistance behaviors from passive to aggressive;
- group resistant behaviors;
- the value of the object or content of resistance;
- the perceived threats to change;
- the internal environment, including power relationships and routines.

More recently, Nilsen et al. (2016) supported the theory of resistance to innovation implementation as being multifaceted and 'expected', existing at the organizational, cultural, technological and ethical level and being a prerequisite to acceptance. This theory is an antithesis to Lewin's theory which considered resistance to change as a barrier to change (Cunningham and Kempling 2009).

We conclude that resistance to change is an expected reaction towards innovation in the healthcare sector, especially from the side of the non-innovators. Resistance to change is also an essential step towards acceptance and adoption of the innovation and it is the leaders' duty to continually motivate the early adopters whilst exploring the behaviours of the non-adopters.

Having a shared vision and purpose amongst organizational teams is the key in moving innovations from early adoption to diffusion stage. The engagement of early adopters (champions) is as valuable exercise as is the late adopter and laggard engagement.

References

Albury D (2005) Fostering innovation in public services. Publ Money Manag

Ash J (1997) Organizational factors that influence information technology diffusion in academic health sciences centers. J Am Med Inform Assoc

Ash JS, Lorenzi NM (2017) Organizational and behavioural issues. In: Key advances in clinical informatics. Chapter 9

Barker PM, Reid A, Schall MW (2016) A framework for scaling up health interventions: lessons from large-scale improvement initiatives in Africa. Implement Sci 11:12

Barlow JG (2013) Strengthening the spread of innovation in the UK's National Health Service. Handbook on innovation in public services. Chapter 35

Barnett J, Vasileiou K, Fayika D et al (2011) Understanding innovators' experience of barriers and facilitators in implementation and diffusion of healthcare service innovations: a qualitative study. BMC Health Serv Res 11(342)

Batt-Rawden KB, Bjork E, Waaler D (2017) Human factors in implementation and adoption of innovations in healthcare services: a longitudinal case study on the introduction of new technology. Innov J 22(3):article 3

Berkhout AJ, Hartmann D, van der Duin P, Ortt R (2006) Innovating the innovation process. Int J Technol Manag 34(3/4):390–404

Berwick DM (2003) Disseminating innovations in healthcare. JAMA 289(15):1969–1975

Bessant J, Tidd J (2013) Managing innovation. www.innovationportal

Birken S, Lee SYD, Weiner BJ (2011) Uncovering middle manager role in healthcare innovation implementation. Implement Sci 7(28)

Bloch C, Bugge M (2013) Public sector innovation–from theory to measurement. Struct Chang Econ Dyn 27:133–145

Blumenthal D, Kilo CM (1998) A report card on continuous innovation: a retro-perspective. Intern J Technol Manag 26(8)

Bourgeois LJ, Brodwin DR (1984) Strategic implementation: five approaches to an elusive phenomenon. Strateg Manag J 5:241–264

Braithwaite J (2018) Changing how we think about healthcare improvement. BMJ 2018(361):k2014

Burnes B (2014) Kurt Lewin and the planned approach to change: a re-appraisal. J Manag Stud 41(6):977–1002

Carreiro H, Oliveira T (2019) Impact of transformational leadership on the diffusion of innovation in firms: Application to mobile cloud computing. Comput Ind 107:104–113

Chen H, Li L and Chen y (2021). Explore success factors that impact artificial intelligence adoption on telecom industry in China. J Manag Anal 8(1):36–68

Chesbrough H, Bogers M (2014) Explicating open innovation: clarifying an emerging paradigm for understanding innovation. In: Chesbrough H, Vanhaverbeke W, West J (eds) New frontiers in open innovation. Oxford University Press, Oxford, pp 3–28

Coetsee L (1999) From resistance to commitment. Public Adm Q 23(2):204–222

Coetsee L (2011) Peak performance and productivity: a practical guide for the creation of a motivating climate. Potchefstroom: Ons drukkers

Collins B (2018) Adoption and spread of innovation in the NHS. The King's Fund

Conner D (2004) White paper. How to be an effective sponsor of major organisational change

Counte MA, Meurer S (2001) Issues in the assessment of continuous quality improvement implementation in healthcare organizations. Int J Qual Healthc 13(3):197–207

Cresswell KM, Cunningham-Burley S, Sheikh A (2016) Creating a climate that catalyses healthcare innovation in the UK—Learning lessons from international innovators. J Innov Health Inform 23(4):772–782

Crompton-Phillips A (2020) Spreading at scale: a practical leadership model for change. NEJM Catalyst 1(1)

Cunningham B, Kempling J (2009) Implementing change in public sector organizations. Manag Decis 47(2):330–344

Currie G, Spyridonidis D (2018) Sharing leadership for diffusion of innovations in professionalised settings. Hum Relat 1–25

Damschroder LJ, Aron DC, Keith RE, Kirsh SR et al (2009) Fostering implementation of health services research findings into practice: a consolidated framework for advancing implementation science. Implement Sci 4:50

Denis JL, Herbert Y, Langley A et al (2002) Explaining diffusion patterns for complex healthcare innovations. Healthc Manag Rev 27(3)

de Ven V (2017) The Innovation journey: you can't control it but you can learn to maneuvre it. Innov Organis Manag 19(1):39–42

Etzkowitz H (2013) Innovation in innovation: the triple helix of university-industry government relations. Soc Sci Inf 42(3):293–337

Ferlie E, Fitzgerald L, Wood M, Hawkins C (2005) Acad Manag J 48(1):117–134

Fleuren M, Wiefferink K, Paulussen T (2004) Determinants of innovation within health care organizations: literature review and Delphi study. Int J Qual Health Care 16(2):107–123

Fukofuka S, Lokke DT (2015) OCTAPACE and organisational resilience: a correlational study. OJBMR 4(1):1–10

Greenhalgh T, Robert G, Macfarlane F et al (2004) Diffusion of innovations in service organizations: systematic review and recommendations. Milbank Q 82(4):581–629

Greenhalgh T, Procter R, Wherton J et al (2012) The organising vision for telehealth and telecare: discourse analysis. MBJ Open 2

Greenhalgh T, Wherton J, Papoutsi C et al (2017) Beyond adoption: a new framework for theorizing and evaluating nonadoption, abandonment and challenges to the scale-up, spread and sustainability of health and care technologies. J Med Internet Res 19(11):e367

Greenhalgh T, Wherton J, Papoutsi C et al (2018) Analysing the role of complexity in explaining the fortunes of technology programmes: empirical application of the NASSS framework. BMC Med 16:66

Helfrich CD, Weiner BJ, McKinney MM, Minasian L (2007) Determinants of implementation effectivenss: adapting a framework of complex innovations. Med Care Res Rev 64(3):279–303

Herscovitch L, Meyer JP (2002) Commitment to organizational change: extension of a three component model. J Appl Psychol 87(3):474–487

Hunter ST, Cushenbery L, Friedrich T (2012) Hiring an Innovative workforce: a necessary yet uniquely challenging endeavor. Hum Resour Manag Rev 22:303–322

Judson A (1999) Changing behavior in organizations: minimizing resistance to change. Blackwell Publishing, Cambridge, MA

Klein KJ, Sorra JS (1996) The challenge of innovation implementation. Acad Manag 21(4):1055–1080

Lapointe L, Rivard S (2005) A multilevel model of resistance to information technology implementation. MIS Q 29(3):461–491

Llewellyn S, Procter R, Harvey G et al (2014) Facilitating technology adoption in the NHS: negotiating the organisational and policy context—A qualitative study. Health Serv Deliv Res 2(23)

Mair FS, May C, O'Donnell C et al (2012) Factors that promote or inhibit the implementation of e-health systems: an explanatory systematic review. Bull World Health Organ 90:357–364

Mani Z, Chouk I (2018) Consumer resistance to innovation in services: challenged and barriers at the internet of things era. J Prod Innov Manag 35(5):763–807

Mannion R, Davies H (2018) Understanding organizational culture for healthcare quality improvement. BMJ 2018(363):k4907

Martin GP, Waring J (2012) Leading from the middle: constrained realities of clinical leadership in healthcare organizations. Health 17(4):358–374

Martins R, Oliveira T, Thomas MA (2016) An empirical analysis to assess the determinants of SaaS diffusion in firms. Comput Hum Behav 62:19–33

May CR, Johnson M, Finch T (2016) Implementation, context and complexity. Implement Sci 11:141

McKee L, Charles K, Dixon-Woods, M et al (2013) New and distributed leadership in quality and safety in healthcare, or old and hierarchical? An interview

Micheli P, Schoeman M, Baxter D, Goffin K (2015) New Business models for public sector innovation. Res Technol Manag 51–57

Mikhailova O (2018) Adoption and implementation of new technologies in hospitals: a network perspective. IMP J 12(2):368–391

Nemeth C, Wears R, Woods D et al (2008) Minding the gaps: creating resilience in healthcare advances in patient safety: new directions and alternative approaches. In: Henriksen K et al (eds) Performance and Tools, vol 3. Agency for Healthcare Research and Quality

Nilsen ER, Dugstad J, Eide H et al (2016) Exploring resistance to implementation of welfare technology in municipal healthcare services—A longitudinal case study. BMC Health Serv Res 16:657

Oke A, Munshi N, Walumbwa MO (2008) The influence of leadership on innovation processes and activities. Organ Dyn 38(1):64–72

Omachonu VK, Einspruch NG (2010) Innovation in healthcare delivery systems: a conceptual framework. Innov J 15(1)

Ovretvbt J, Scott T, Rundall T et al (2007) Improving quality through effective implementation of information technology in healthcare. Int J Qual Healthc 19(5):259–266

Pryor MG, Anderson D, Toombs L, Humphreys JH (2007) Strategic implementation as a core competency. J Manag Res 7(1)

Ranga M, Etzkowitz H (2013) Triple Helix systems: an analytical framework for innovation policy and practice in the knowledge society. Ind High Educ 27(3):237–262

Rogers EM (1995) Diffusion of innovations, 4th edn. Free Press, New York

Ross J, Stevenson F, Lau R, Murray E (2016) Factors that influence the implementation of e-health: a systematic review of systematic reviews. Implement Sci 11:146

Sahin I (2006) Detailed review of Rogers' diffusion of innovations theory and educational technology-related studies based on Roger's theory. Turkish Online J Edu Technol 5(2):article 3

Social Care Institute for Excellence (2018) Leadership in integrated health systems. Fut Care (9)

Valente TW, Davis RL (1995). Accelerating the diffusion of innovations using opinion leaders. Annals AAPSS 565

Valente TW, Pumpuang P (2007) Identifying opinion leaders to promote behaviour change. Health Educ Behav 34(6):881–896

Van Gemert-Pijnen J, Nijland N, van Limburg M et al (2011) A holistic framework to improve the uptake and impact of eHealth technologies. J Med Internet Res 13(4):e111

Van Limburg M, van Gemert-Pijnen J, Seydel ER (2011) Why business modelling is crucial in the development of eHealth technologies. J Med Internet Res 13(4):e124

Verna JY, Rossiter M, Kirvan K et al (2013) Going far together: healthcare collaborations for innovation and improvement in Canada. Int J Healthc Manag 6(2)

Waldman DA, Bass BM (1991) Transformational leadership at different phases of the innovation process. J High Technol Manag Res 2(2):169–180

Wani TA, Ali SW (2015) Innovation diffusion theory. J Gener Manag Res 3(2):101–118

Weintraub P, McKee M (2019) Leadeship for innovation in healthcare: an exploration. Int J Health Policy Manag 3:138–144

West MA (2002) Sparkling fountains or stagnant ponds: an integrative model of creativity and innovation implementation in work groups. Appl Psychol: Int Rev 51(3):355–424

Yang Z, Sun J, Zhang Y, Wang Y (2015) Understanding SaaS adoption from the perspective of organizational users: a tripod readiness model. Comput Hum Behav 45:254–264

3

Learning from Innovation Failure—*A Case Study*

Abstract The first innovation case study is a linear innovation process in the NHS that began with a clinical innovator and front-line clinician generating an idea. The idea was shared with the Trust innovation senior forum and was supported by the Trust 's executive team. The innovator partnered with key stakeholders in order to compete for a national funding innovation competition process, which would enable the innovator to move the idea into the adoption and piloting phase. The opportunity for diffusion and scale up of innovation depended primarily on the initial adoption phase and secondarily on the resources of the organization. Resources that were identified as essential for building the innovation included information technology system interfacing, data migration, Apps and other digital architectural capabilities. Commercial and marketing capabilities were also essential for the Trust to scale up the innovation. The clinical innovator was unsuccessful in securing the national funding for the pilot and the innovation stalled at the pre-adoption stage. The case elaborates on the enablers and barriers to innovation adoption from a leadership perspective and also touches upon leadership aspects of innovation diffusion, implementation and scale up which need to be considered when planning the adoption of innovation.

3.1 Idea Generation

The innovator, a senior clinician in the healthcare organization under study, proposed the idea of a remote monitoring digital solution for cancer patients undergoing chemotherapy, which would enable patients to report their symptoms to their clinical team remotely. By doing so, patients would alert their acute oncology clinical team to signs of clinical deterioration warranting urgent review leading to prevention of patient deterioration and hospital admission avoidance. An internal organizational audit led by the innovator, revealed that 30% of cancer patients on chemotherapy admitted to hospital with fever, could have been managed in the community, if patients had access to a remote monitoring tool to be able to report their symptoms directly to their clinical team. The audit results generated the innovation idea, which was subsequently worked up to a formal innovation proposal.

> Being admitted into Accident and Emergency with complications of chemotherapy is often worse than the chemotherapy itself; very stressful for the individual and the family; the hospital is a scary place when you have no control of what's going on with you
>
> **Cancer patient carer**

The purpose of the innovation was to provide cancer patients undergoing chemotherapy with a user-friendly and modern digital communication tool to be able to report their symptoms to their acute oncology clinical teams and get prompt advice directly without the need to visit the hospital or clinic. The communication platform would be done through a patient portal and it would enable the creation of an organised database comprising of:

(1) patient symptoms (input from patients);
(2) clinical advice (acute oncology intervention) and
(3) patient outcomes (output).

The patient outcomes could range from self-management information (Green), outpatient clinic attendance in 24 h (Amber) or admission to accident and emergency (Red). Overtime and with the growth of data, the innovation team could train a chatbot on the algorithm (input − intervention − outcome) using machine-learning and natural language processing.

The creation of a chatbot which would sit within the patient portal, would give the most appropriate advice to patients, rather than utilising a member of staff to do this. The chatbot would eventually become the communication platform that sits within the patient portal and with which patients would interact. This would free up time for the acute oncology teams to look after sick patients who are already in the hospital.

The innovation idea was generated by a single clinician innovator, following the production of local evidence of need and an extensive literature review of the evidence of remote patient monitoring in healthcare. The proposed benefits of the innovation that were drawn from the local audit and the literature review were the following:

- To reduce unplanned admissions of oncology patients receiving chemotherapy.
- To reduce Emergency department attendance of oncology patients receiving chemotherapy.
- To extend survival time of oncology patients (no sepsis deaths).
- To improve compliance with chemotherapy treatment.
- To reduce non-attendance rates for clinics and tests.
- To empower and activate patients to participate in their disease management.
- To improve quality of patient care and experience particularly in terms of health care provider responsiveness to chemotherapy related patient problems.

The stakeholders impacted were the following:

Patients—no unnecessary admissions, increased trust in service, improved self-management, reduction in time spent trying to engage with service, more efficient chemotherapy provision, no travel time and costs, removal of need to take time of work to physically attend, no parking costs, no time wasted for relative or carer.

Patient/family/carers—reduced anxiety about when to engage with hospital, easier to make contact and reduction in time trying to engage with service.

Oncology clinical team—possibly increased workload at weekends; reduced burnout as job less frustrating; overtime, more remote working rather than physical review of patients on the wards or the emergency department.

Emergency department—reduced contacts with chemotherapy patients and improved flow.

Hospital wards receiving admissions—reduced unnecessary admissions of chemotherapy patients.

Pharmacy at hospital—reduced wastage of systemic anticancer drug therapy, as any changes to treatment can be predicted.

Hospital overall—released resources that can be used for improving quality of care, reduction in footfall through the hospital, less congestion on site parking, freeing up clinic room capacity, potential reduction of clinic non-attendance rates.

Cancer patient representatives found the idea of a digital platform positive for managing their cancer better. Their views were sought through two patient and public engagement events. There was general agreement amongst cancer patients that the platform provided opportunities to enhance existing cancer services.

> I value the opportunity to have virtual contact with my doctor or nurse between clinic appointments and have my symptoms dealt with in a timely manner, rather than waiting until the next clinical appointment
>
> **Cancer Patient 1**

Patient insights helped the digital innovation team understand what excellence looks and feels like for patients, what aspects of the existing services are important to them and several ways the digital innovation could improve existing services. Being able to keep track of their appointment schedule virtually, having access to their clinical team between clinical appointments and having the option of a virtual clinic through their mobile phone, were highly valued. In fact, evidence from the LYNC digital study (Griffiths et al. 2017) suggests that digital technologies can help reduce intrusion of cancer treatment into people's daily routines, as patients can check appointments remotely and contact their clinical team as required.

> The technology should be personalised and easy to use; a good mix of patients, some technologically savvy and some not should be involved in the implementation process
> **Cancer patient 2**

> Remote access to my own treatment plan diary would be very helpful, it would remind me of my clinic appointments and all the tests and treatments I need to attend to so as not to miss any
> **Cancer patient 3**

> The technology has the potential to improve speed of access to doctor advice and spare me unnecessary trips to the hospital, this is really powerful
> **Cancer patient 4**

> The ability to have my clinic consultation online would give me the opportunity to see the doctor from the comfort of my own home and my wife who is disabled can attend also
> **Cancer patient 5**

The innovator was convinced that the idea was viable and could help patients and the organization in multiple ways, so proceeded in putting the idea forward for consideration at the organization's Ideas Den. The innovator's idea was shortlisted and the innovator was invited to present at the Ideas Den.

3.2 The Ideas Den

The innovator was the first to ever present an innovation idea at the Ideas Den. The purpose of the Ideas Den was for the Trust executives to prioritize innovations based on clinical and organizational value.

> The 'Ideas Den' is a great initiative to enable front line innovators to share their ideas and compete for the chance to receive resources, which would support them to develop and implement their innovation
> **NHS Organization Executive 1**

The Innovation and Transformation teams had received the Trust's commitment to support the implementation of the shortlisted innovations in terms of offering industry partnerships, dedicated project management support and funding to build innovations that would add value to the organization.

> It is expected that the Trust will invest in the best innovation ideas voted by the Den, that's the whole purpose of it
> **Innovation Manager**

At the Idea's Den, the Executives and non-Executive Directors got interested in the proposed digital innovation which they subsequently shortlisted, because of its perceived value.

In order to strengthen the case for adoption of this innovation, the researcher and innovator presented a study from the Memorian Sloan Kettering Hospital to the Ideas Den, which demonstrated the value of remote patient monitoring in Oncology, as applied in a different healthcare system. In specific, the study revealed that if cancer patients reported their symptoms to their clinical teams during and between chemotherapy treatments through the use of remote monitoring tools, they lived 5.2 months longer than patients who didn't (Basch et al. 2017).

The innovator also presented the internal audit outcomes and the published quantitative and qualitative evidence of the innovation. Similar benefits have been documented in the literature about clinical specialties other than Oncology, such as cardiology, diabetes and respiratory medicine (COPD). The presence of such comprehensive evidence on the value of the innovation, validated its proof of concept and convinced the Ideas Den that the innovation would be something valuable to apply in the organization.

The vision of the innovator was the adoption and diffusion of the remote monitoring model of care in all Oncological specialties within the organization. In addition, if the model proved successful in Oncology, it could be scaled up across other medical specialties (rheumatology, hematology, pediatrics) as well as other organizations. The benefit realization plan from scaling up such innovation in the NHS, in terms of improving patient safety and patient experience whilst reducing healthcare costs, was the attractive factor in the Ideas Den innovation selection process.

The innovator transferred knowledge to the Den from the existing pool of quantitative and qualitative evidence of similar innovations in same and different healthcare systems and also supplemented such knowledge with data that were applicable to the organization, which demonstrated value to the organization and beyond. The innovator used local, national and international data to increase buy-in from the hospital senior management team, in order for them to endorse the innovation. The same tactic was subsequently used to engage other front-line clinical leaders. By doing so, the innovator maximized the chances of local innovation adoption which would enable the effectiveness of the innovation.

A successful adoption pilot study, accompanied by the evaluation of pilot outcomes in terms of quantitative and qualitative outcomes, would support the innovation being diffused to other clinical specialties within the organization. This is in line with the theory of innovation adoption and diffusion supported by Ferlie et al. (2005) and Barnett et al. (2011), who explored the views of front-line clinical leaders and found that the presence of quantitative evidence could make innovations more likely to diffuse.

3.3 The Innovation Team

The innovator, a front-line senior doctor, led a team of 14 people from within and outside the organization, in the preparation of the innovation bid for the purpose of receiving funding to pilot the innovation. The patient portal would integrate with the existing oncology electronic health record which captured all patient demographics and treatment details.

> Remote patient monitoring is utilized to enable patient schedule their appointments more efficiently and also gain access to their records; the innovation team will exploit all capabilities of the portal including interacting with patients and proactively managing their condition which will translate to better cancer patient outcomes
> **Portal vendor**

The innovation project plan included the co-design of the patient portal functionalities with the support of cancer patients and clinicians, in order to meet the needs of the desired care model. The interfacing between the portal and the oncology health record meant that the full repository of clinical information about cancer patient visits, test results and clinical outcomes could be securely shared between patients and their clinical teams. The addition of a conversational platform (chatbot) represented an additional disruptive innovation to the proposed remote patient monitoring model of care.

> The addition of the bot onto a patient portal which integrates with the patient health care record, the latter used by 50% of the cancer hospitals and clinics nationally and internationally, gives the innovation its unique service proposition and makes the innovation scalable and sustainable
> **NHS Senior radiographer 1**

The benefit realization plan of the innovation would be measured following the innovation launch and various parameters would be measured 6-monthly for the first year and then yearly thereafter and until year 5. Financial benefit realization included the return on investment (ROI) in terms of cost efficiencies achieved from the reduction of hospital admissions and length of stay, reduction of outpatient clinic appointments, non-attendances in clinic and lost to follow up costs. In addition, pharmacy waste would be reduced due to the prompt alteration of the chemotherapy regime when needed.

> If we know early that a patient is not well enough to attend next chemotherapy cycle, we could offer the treatment space to another patient and pharmacy staff would not waste any expensive chemotherapy drugs on the day because of patient non-attendance
> **NHS chemotherapy senior nurse**

Non-financial benefit realization included the improvement in patient quality of life, reduction in mortality and morbidity from chemotherapy complications, improvement in patient and staff experience.

> The patient experience with patient portal will determine if patients continue to use it, so clinical teams operating the portal need to be responsive from its launch
>
> **Academic partner**

When putting the business case together for the bid, most of the innovation costs were due to the patient portal license and the integration between the portal and the oncology electronic health record. This integration required investment from the Trust in terms of expert time and also commitment from the Trust, in terms of maintaining the innovation beyond the adoption pilot.

However, following the Ideas Den's approval of the innovation, it became apparent that the organizational budget could not support the license costs for the patient portal. In addition, the internal organizational infrastructure could not support the integration between the portal and the oncology health record.

> There are not enough technical people in the organization to support this innovation without delaying or disinvesting in other projects
>
> **Lead IT architect**

After discussions between the innovator and the hospital management teams, it became apparent that the execution of the system integration required specialist IT workforce time which was not included in the Trust budget for the financial year. As a result, the innovator's expectations of an organizational support for the implementation of the innovation, did not actually materialize. Despite the fact that innovation benefits would be realized within the first 3 years of the innovation deployment including an ROI of 20% at year 3 of deployment, the Trust was not prepared to invest financial and workforce resources for the deployment of this technology.

> The organization runs on a deficit and there are no funds to support Apps or other digital development from scratch; all investment on digital technologies needs to be devoted to the procurement on the future Trust-wide Electronic Health Record
> **NHS Organization Executive 2**

Another reason behind the organizational reluctance to invest in a remote patient monitoring system at the time, was the Trust strategic plan to acquire a Trust-wide Electronic Health Record (EHR) system in the near future, which would include a patient portal as well. This made the proposed integration cost look wasteful.

Although the innovator and the organization shared the same vision for a remote patient monitoring model of care for all outpatient medical specialties, there were barriers to the implementation of such model of care, as described below:

- the lack of funding for the purchasing of the patient portal;
- the lack of internal IT workforce capacity and expertise;
- the cost of system interfacing between the portal and the oncology EHR;
- future plans to purchase a Trust-wide EHR including its own portal, despite deployment timelines being unclear at the time

Despite those innovation barriers, the Ideas Den approved the innovator's proposal and gave the 'go-ahead' to the innovator to prepare for submission to a national innovation funding competition. The external funding would cover the purchase of the portal for 18 months (adoption pilot), the integration costs including workforce time and the evaluation of implementation piece, for a total time of 18 months. The latter was suggested as the proposed timeline for this innovation to become adopted and diffused within the oncology specialties.

There was an ethical dilemma as to what would happen to the innovation once the external funding finished and whether the Trust would be in a different financial position and be prepared to fund the portal license and support the integration maintenance or whether the innovation technology would stop altogether.

> It is concerning to think that an innovation which proves to be beneficial to patients gets withdrawn after the end of the pilot period
> **Research & Development staff member**

For the purpose of the innovation fund competition submission, the innovator together with an IT project manager, co-chaired an innovation steering committee, the members of which were as follows:

- The clinical innovator, key opinion leader and sponsor of the project
- An NHS IT project manager
- Two senior therapeutic radiographers and oncology EHR experts
- Two senior NHS acute oncology nurses
- A lead IT architect from the NHS organization

- An academic professor with previous experience on leading remote monitoring studies, who led on the evaluation of implementation
- Two commercial business partners
- An NHS commercial lead responsible for intellectual property
- A member of the academic health science network who led on the patient and public involvement element of the program
- A member of the Research and Development team
- A research fellow from the local university who observed the innovation process from a leadership perspective.

The committee met on a weekly basis between January 2018 and July 2018, the duration of the Innovate UK application process, in order to monitor performance and ensure stakeholder actions were delivered on time. Meetings were well attended and resulted in the timely completion of both stages in the application process.

> The culture of the meetings was collaborative and inclusive and there was good leadership throughout
> **Academic fellow**

The innovator engaged with the academic partner in the first instance given her previous work on remote monitoring in young adults with chronic illnesses (Griffiths et al. 2017). The collaboration between the academic partner, the vendor of the portal and the bot partner was strengthened by further engagement meetings which the innovator led. It was important that the three external partners to the organization had a trusting relationship with each other and were aligned with the vision of the organization. Building a strong relationship between the NHS organization and the three partners was important to the innovator who looked at the bigger picture and beyond the 18-month project; the innovator's vision was the diffusion and scale up of remote patient monitoring in the NHS and the provision of sustainable teams who would deliver this.

Interorganizational partnerships are key for the successful adoption and diffusion of innovations (Barnett et al. 2011). The collaboration between industry, academia and government organizations is key in maximizing innovation success (Nilsen et al. 2016). However, cultural differences between industry and academia may sometimes compromise user acceptance by compromising the communication of innovation outcomes to end users (Lundvall 2016). In the digital innovation case, there were conflicted interests amongst the various partners which the innovator attempted to iron out for the purpose of delivering on their common goal which was the digital technology implementation.

3.4 Stakeholder Engagement and The Evaluation Process

Prior to the final grant submission, the innovator led two patient and public involvement (PPI) group forums, where patients had the chance to comment on the digital innovation concept and functionalities from a patient and end-user perspective. Their response was positive and supportive regardless of their age which ranged between 40 and 75 years old. The innovator's concern was that elderly patients would find the digital tool impractical, but this was not the case.

> I would have liked to be able to reach my clinical team and let them know how I felt in-between my clinic appointments; the portal would enable me to do that and I would use it for that purpose
>
> **Patient 6**

> I am a bit old-fashioned and I want to see my doctor face to face; saying that, it feels isolating when you only see them every 3 weeks; the portal is good for some people but not for me, I would like to be able to speak to the doctor on the phone instead
>
> **Patient 7**

Although there was strong support from the majority of patient representatives, it was clear that the innovation team had to provide for patients who wouldn't be able or wouldn't want to use the digital technology. Digital exclusion was a risk and therefore ensuring that patients also had access to the clinical team on the phone rather than just the portal—chatbot interaction, was extremely important.

The academic partner who recruited the evaluation team had already published extensively around digital communication tools for young people living with long term conditions (Griffiths et al. 2017). There was strong evidence already published about the fact that timely digital communication between chronically ill patients and their care provider improves engagement with health care, empowers patients and activates them to self-manage their health concerns (Griffiths et al. 2017). Again, the provision of the standard service for patients who wouldn't use digital technology was key.

The academic partner and her team would lead the evaluation of the innovation implementation which included service use data and interviews with all innovation stakeholders including patients. The data collection would be around the acceptability of the innovation, barriers and enablers, as well as the perceived impact of the innovation. The evaluation was planned to start early in the innovation process and as soon as funding became available. By doing so, the evaluation would capture the engagement aspect with end users, the recruitment of participants and the end to end experience of patients, staff and carers.

The objectives of the evaluation from an end user perspective were the following:

- Understanding user experience of the intervention from the patient and carer's perspectives;
- Measuring the use of innovation features by patients and the acute oncology team;
- Evaluating which patients use/do not use the intervention and understand whether the intervention changes equality of access;
- Understanding from the perspective of the acute oncology team how the intervention is implemented, barriers and facilitators to implementation and how they are overcome and the experience of using the intervention;
- Assessing the impact of the intervention on patient pathway compliance, A&E attendance and unplanned admissions;
- Costing the innovation and estimating its cost-effectiveness compared with current practice in reducing A&E attendance rates, mortality rate within 30 days of cancer treatment, unplanned hospital admissions and inpatient length of stay, whilst improving treatment compliance;
- Compare clinical team and Artificial Intelligence (AI) based decision-making (chatbot);
- Explore the social and ethical implications of the use of AI;
- Health economics to evaluate the economic impact of the service.

The success of innovation projects, as with any change management process, is highly dependent on the degree of end user acceptance of the innovation (Dillon and Morris 1996). An approach to innovation adoption and diffusion similar to Taylor's autocratic management theory, whereby employees follow their director's orders and focus only on performance, is unlikely to fit well in today's competitive organizational environments (Martinez-Cardoso 2014). Studies of user involvement in medical device innovation have shown that users have to be involved at different stages in the medical device lifecycle including scoping, validation, design and evaluation (Money et al. 2011). In case of the digital innovation in the NHS, end user involvement in the design and implementation of the innovation would ensure that it meets user needs and that any changes would be justified and driven by end users (Vincent and Blandford 2011). There were two main end users in this case, patients and NHS staff. Carers were also included, especially if patients were relying on carers to use the innovation. The evaluation of the implementation would include all end user experience.

Although the external environment may stimulate the decision to innovate, the internal organizational leadership and culture plays an important role in the adoption, implementation and diffusion of innovations. In particular, the attitude towards innovation from organizational leaders, their influential and motivational skills and the degree to which they include staff and other end users, determines the success or failure of innovation (Damanpour and Schneider 2006). There are clear strategic, quality, cost and operational benefits from user involvement early on and throughout the innovation process (Shah and Robinson 2007), including leveraging user experience and knowledge in improving innovation functionalities and reducing costs. Early user involvement can validate the innovation and offer some security that the innovation is likely to be adopted if other stakeholder factors are met.

In this NHS innovation case study, early patient user involvement validated the proposed innovation as a viable and effective means of patient-clinician interaction with clear patient and organizational benefits.

Patient-public involvement (PPI) in the early scoping stage of the innovation process was perceived as an important component of the project by the Innovate UK panel. On the other hand, the lack of a wider clinician network involvement including Oncology doctors, GPs and commissioners in the early stages of the project was seen negatively, because it did not support the scalability of the innovation. Similar engagement work to the PPI work should have been done with internal medical staff as well as external stakeholders (GPs and commissioners) in order to maximize user acceptance. Other staff such as nurses and radiographers were receptive to the idea and its implementation and were engaged well from the start, unlike medical staff and external stakeholders.

Unlike oncology nursing staff who were supportive of the innovation and engaged early on during the conception of the innovation, there was significant resistance to the innovation idea from the rest of the oncology clinicians (the non-innovators). The resistance came primarily from the perceived increased workload, which trumped any enthusiasm around the innovation. Exploring the resistant behaviour a bit more, it became apparent that a mobile application was piloted few years previously to try and engage patients remotely but the latter failed to be adopted. It transpired that the remote monitoring device which was piloted in the past, was not as intuitive as the proposed innovation. In addition, the threshold for patients contacting the clinical team was set too low which meant that patients were calling the clinical teams unnecessarily (false alarms). This created more waste in terms of workforce time.

> We have piloted this before and it didn't work; it was a disaster, as patients kept ringing us based on the traffic light system on the App but there was no clinical reason to ring; this new system would not work either and we have so much work to do anyway
> **Consultant Oncologist 1**

Once the previous innovation technology was abandoned, clinicians lost confidence to digital remote monitoring technologies. As a result, they were reluctant to pilot the proposed innovation. In the long term, the innovation would likely reduce clinician workload, due to fewer hospital admissions and fewer outpatient clinics. In the short-term and during the pilot phase, the innovation would likely be set to be risk-averse and ensure that patients who needed advice got hold of their clinical team straight away. By doing so, doctors' workload would be expected to go up initially as they would be responding to more patient calls. Eventually, the doctors' workload would reduce as end users would gain more confidence in the chatbot system.

The oncology doctors resisted the change from current model of care to the remote model, despite the presentation by the innovator of short-term and long-term benefits for patients, the organization and staff. The innovator failed to attract a second doctor to co-lead the innovation steering group as a result. The perceived lack of usefulness of the innovation by the doctors and the unwillingness to pilot the technology meant that the innovator had no support from peers.

There was also an element of power difference and control between the innovator and the non-innovators. The past attempt by another clinical innovator within the department to design and implement a similar technology failed to be adopted beyond a small pilot. The decision of the oncology doctors not to support the current more refined idea may have been influenced by the past failure, as a means of being loyal to the previous innovator. The lack of support may also be explained by a somewhat antagonistic behaviour amongst clinicians. The lack of available funding and clinician disinterest in developing the past digital technology further, may have led to the lack of clinician support. An attempt by the clinical innovator to secure some funding from the charitable funds by engaging fellow clinicians in the oncology department also met with lack of support.

> We didn't progress the 'old' innovation and that was a unanimous decision, so why should we support the same innovation two years later
>
> **Consultant Oncologist 2**

The lack of clinician engagement was viewed negatively by the external innovation fund committee panel, in terms of hindering the innovation adoption and diffusion process.

3.5 The Final Decision About Innovation Adoption

The national innovation panel interviewed the project team in August 2018 and scored the innovation favourably in terms of fulfilling an important gap in clinical care of cancer patients. The innovation offered tangible benefits to the Trust and the local community, adding value through patient pathway efficiencies, better patient experience and improvement in clinical outcomes (prevention of deteriorating patient and reducing mortality and morbidity from chemotherapy).

The judges supported the fact that the team run two successful patient and public involvement forums and received positive feedback from patients who perceived the technology to be useful for them. Although the project team were not the final winners of the innovation fund award, they came very close to be awarded.

The main reason for the decision of commissioners not to allocate the fund to this innovation, was the lack of a robust strategic plan to diffuse the innovation beyond the local NHS and scale it up to other NHS organizations. In addition, the lack of an organised engagement plan with the local clinical commissioning group (CCG) meant that the innovation team had not considered a system-wide implementation of the innovation which would support its diffusion and sustainability.

Moreover, the panel had concerns regarding the business leadership and commercial capability of the organization at the time. They identified a risk in the technical implementation of the innovation, as well as the ability of the organization to sustain the innovation beyond the funding period. Given that the benefit realization plan was so compelling, it almost felt unethical to set up a remote patient monitoring model of care and then withdraw the model once the pilot period ended.

Furthermore, the panel commented on the patients less able to possess or utilise digital technology who would be potentially excluded from the service. This would create health inequalities in the access of care for oncology patients. The concerns were addressed well by the team who presented a clear action plan about keeping current process whilst improving digital literacy of patients.

Finally, the panel were concerned about the lack of internal peer support for the innovator. Without clinical doctor support, it would be difficult for the innovation to be diffused and sustained.

One of the reviewer comments was the following:

> There is a concern about less able patients, or patients with mild cognitive impairment (MCI) and dementia accessing the technology
>
> **Commissioner 1**

The innovation team response to this comment was the following:

> We will work closely with our patient partners to ensure that our methods for data collection are appropriate
>
> Patient information within the portal is written at a 9th grade level. Where possible, we will provide support for patients in participating. The clinical staff involved in the project, are all trained to work with less mentally able patients. Those patients are in any case selected carefully by their clinical team for chemotherapy treatment
>
> **Patient and Public Involvement lead**

Another comment by the Innovation Panel around the sustainability of the innovation was the following:

> There is no clear strategic plan of how the innovation will be scaled up and sustained; a discussion with the local clinical commissioning group to secure their support would have been reassuring
>
> **Commissioner 2**

The decision of the innovation commissioners not to fund the innovation was disappointing for the innovation team, especially as the innovation commissioners recognised and verbalised the positive value of the innovation for patients, the organization and the community. The team took on board the feedback from the commissioners and met together in order to reflect and make plans forward. The dedication of the leadership team and their belief in the innovation benefits led them to look for alternative funding streams.

3.6 Lessons on Leadership

The organization's executive team's intent to support frontline clinical innovators was the correct one but 'innovation' was not included in the budget plan and therefore not adequately invested on. There was no innovation strategy, no vision or roadmap for innovation and no innovation deliverables defined within the organization.

The innovation and transformation teams were managed by motivated and engaged managers but they lacked clinical leadership within the teams. This made the clinician engagement for innovation adoption difficult across the Trust. In addition, the research and development (R&D) department worked independently from the innovation and transformation departments, which made it more difficult to leverage the R&D resources for innovation.

The innovation already had proven value through trial-based clinical outcomes, this is a prerequisite for innovation adoption according to Rogers (1995), Barnett et al. (2011) and Greenhalgh (2018). The remote monitoring model of care proposed through this innovation, had led to a 45% reduction in cancer patient mortality in one study based in U.S (Newman et al. 2011). In another study conducted at the Institute Inter-régional de Cancérologie Jean Bernard in Le Mans, in France, advanced lung-cancer patients were randomized between remote symptom monitoring through a smartphone App and standard care. The patients who submitted weekly symptom reports to their doctors via the app lived significantly longer (75% vs 49% at 1 year) (Winslow 2016). Basch et al. (2017) showed in their randomized study of 766 cancer patients, that those patients who were monitored remotely for symptoms during their treatment, had >5 months improved survival than the controls. This level of survival advantage is comparable to phase III drug therapy trials, but the cost of this approach is significantly less than drug costs (Basch et al. 2017).

The evidence behind this digital innovation in terms of improving clinical outcomes for cancer patients was the key value proposition for patients and the organization. Further evidence around remote cancer patient monitoring systems suggested a 15% reduction in Accident and Emergency visits through proactive symptom management, a 20% reduction in emergency admissions, a 14% reduction in elective admissions, a 14% reduction in bed days and an 8% reduction in tariff costs (Newman et al. 2011).

Cancer patients could be better managed in the community, offering significant savings for the NHS and with significantly scalable cost-saving potential. The digital innovation proposal would enable that. However, the organization lacked innovation readiness capabilities and leadership for innovation (Greenhalgh et al. 2018). The lack of organizational resilience in terms of having the resources, early adopters, clinical champions (the doctors) and executive leadership for innovation, were key factors in the failure to adopt this innovation. A reflection on the lack of doctor engagement and support may also be due to the lack of a wider organizational response to innovation calls by front-line clinicians.

The innovator engaged business partners with proven track record of successful implementations in large hospitals and with commercial and marketing capabilities which is a positive element in innovation diffusion success (Etzkowitz 2013; Omachonu and Einspruch 2010). However, what the organization lacked at the time was the technical, digital architectural and the commercial expertise to be able to implement the innovation. The lack of technical and commercial capabilities resulted in the innovation commissioner losing confidence in the spread and sustainability of the innovation beyond the pilot stage.

The presence of the business partners and their engagement by the clinical innovator played a very important role in the innovation being shortlisted by the commissioners. However, the relationship between the NHS and the two separate business partners as well as the academic partner, posed some complexity when it came to the ownership of the innovation and future risk sharing. This made it difficult for other commercial partners to invest on the innovation following the failure to secure the innovation fund.

Apart from a single clinical champion and sponsor of the innovation and a dedicated project team, there was lack of key stakeholder engagement (Etzkowitz 2013; Chesbrough and Bogers 2014) in the innovation. On a positive leadership note, the clinical innovator applied open Innovation principles, through the creation of external partnerships to the NHS organization, including academic institutions and the commercial sector. The champion and sponsor of the innovation (the clinical innovator) drove the knowledge sharing and partner engagement for the purpose of innovation acceleration. The innovator acted as a knowledge broker, engaging with clinicians, patients and other end users in order to apply evidence into clinical practice.

However, the clinical innovator should have performed a more detailed stakeholder analysis to understand the power and influence of all stakeholders in driving the proposed innovation forward. The failure to perform this activity resulted in GPs and the CCG being left out from the engagement process. As a result of the lack of broader stakeholder endorsement, the innovation commissioners were not sufficiently reassured that the organization could diffuse and scale the innovation beyond the initial adoption phase.

An academic fellow conducted an independent evaluation of a number of innovation processes in the NHS Trust under study, including our digital innovation process. The findings of his study demonstrated the key role of clinical as well as organizational leadership in driving the adoption and diffusion of innovation. He commented on the important role of the organization's innovation department in engaging clinical innovators and enabling them to act as knowledge brokers within the Trust. The purpose of the innovation department was to act autonomously, attracting innovators to come forward with their innovative ideas and being able to compete for organizational resources. At the same time, the organization leaders should honour their commitment to support the innovators with the necessary resources for them to implement and scale their innovations. The innovation and transformation departments acted as facilitators and as the link between clinical innovators, academics and the industry, supporting innovators with grant applications and intellectual property. However, it transpired that the innovation department could not act autonomously as it did not have the funds to support the procurement of digital technology or the mobilisation and allocation of workforce resources.

The fact that many different innovation ideas within the same organization stalled early in the process, was attributed to the lack of organizational resources in supporting the adoption and diffusion of innovations. The innovation and transformation departments were linked to the research and development department when it came to grant applications, but otherwise, their activities were independent. For example, research funds from clinical trials within the Trust were not shared with the innovation department. In addition, the innovation department performance was not measured against any indicators, unlike the research and development department.

The lack of autonomy and resources in the innovation department to support the implementation of valuable innovations, shows the lack of organisational resilience with regards to innovation at the time (Fukofuka and Lokke 2015). The lack of investment in the innovation department posed a risk, in that clinical innovators could stop coming forward with ideas or could find other means to develop their innovations, often outside the organization.

A significant leadership barrier to this digital innovation succeeding, was the oncology doctor stance (the non-innovators), who were unsupportive of the innovation being piloted. The perception of complexity and low value of the innovation by the rest of the oncology doctors, who would have been the end users of the innovation, posed a threat to the success of the adoption pilot. The reason behind the doctors' resistance to support the digital innovation was the concern that it would potentially require significant time investment from them and that it would increase their daily workload. Clinicians were also concerned that patients and clinicians needed to be trained to use the technology and such model of care did not form part of their standard clinical practice. There was also an element of mistrust in the digital technology given poor experience with a similar technology in the past. Moreover, power differences between innovator and non-innovators may have played a role in the decision not to adopt the innovation. The ownership of innovation fell on the clinical innovator who sought support from peers in making it happen. A similar innovation whose pilot was unsuccessful took place some years before and was led by another clinician in the oncology department. That might have influenced the willingness to support the new innovation. Finally, there was an element of mistrust on the organizational capabilities to support and invest on innovation which may have led to doctor disengagement.

> No clear evidence to change my clinical practice
> **Consultant Oncologist 3**

> I can see the benefit to patients straight away and long-term will have a huge impact in the way we care for patients, but requires significant consultant buy-in to the new model of care for this to succeed.
> **Acute Oncology nurse**

> Standardisation of data collection is a prerequisite for the chatbot to succeed and this needs doctor engagement; variable quality of data collection would make the vision of an AI-based advisory tool non-attainable
> **NHS Senior radiographer 2**

> There is no time for me to spend innovating, as there is no remuneration associated with it and only the Trust will benefit
> **Consultant Oncologist 4**

We have identified some organisational issues that might have led to the non-adoption of the innovation:

- The organization did not have funding, workforce resources or the industrial relations to support this digital innovation project either as a pilot or beyond the funded pilot stage. The organization's limited technical and commercial capabilities made the project 'high risk' in terms of its sustainability after the funded pilot.
- The organization lacked a culture of experimentation and risk-taking which was perceived as a lack of organizational support amongst clinicians and other internal and external stakeholders. There was also no strategy for innovation across the organization and as a healthcare system.
- There was a degree of misalignment between the organization's vision to promote innovation and the resources available for innovation execution.
- There was a perceived lack of a coalition between the organization's innovation department and its Research and Development department, which meant that any innovation project being proposed by the innovation department was not necessarily backed up by the organization's R&D infrastructure and resources.
- There was lack of a structured engagement strategy between the commissioners and the organization when it came to innovation, despite the fact that commissioners would be required to support the diffusion of innovations.

If the Trust wants clinical innovators to continue to come forward with improvement and disruptive ideas that can have a financial and quality value for the Trust, it needs to invest on innovation resources to support front-line innovators, otherwise these people will leave us
NHS innovation manager

Deep diving into the barriers to innovation adoption in this case, we also identified the lack of protected clinician time for innovation work. In addition to that, there was lack of clinician incentivization in terms of time, space and pay to encourage innovation. Clinician incentivization was deemed to be an important factor for clinical leader motivation to lead on innovation. There was lack of protected time in the clinician job plan for innovation work, lack of sessional pay for innovation and recognition of the work clinicians were prepared to put in to making innovation happen. Moreover, there were few or no opportunities for networking with other innovation leaders across the country or with the industry and no opportunities for promotion. Adding to the above disincentives, there was resistance from doctors to adopt a new technology even as a pilot, because it could potentially alter the routine work structure and introduce significant change to the department.

In summary the innovation project could positively improve the model of cancer care delivered in the NHS Trust but stalled before the adoption stage, primarily due to lack of funding and secondarily due to lack of organizational readiness for innovation. Even if the innovation grant was awarded, the innovation would have stalled after the initial pilot, because there was no strategic approach to innovation adoption and diffusion.

Following the unsuccessful innovation bid and given that the Trust had no funding to support the project, the innovator had three choices:

- to drop the idea;
- to seek alternative funding sources;
- to re-apply for the innovation after addressing panel's comments.

The idea was finally dropped which led to members of the innovation and transformation teams leaving the organization for other external roles.

The discussion that was held with those people revealed a consistent message as to what drove them to pursue roles outside the organization:

- the complexity of the NHS meant that there was an urgent need for innovation and change, but the consistent lack of resources for innovation, led to conflict between vision and reality;
- the poor business capabilities of the organization and the competition for limited resources, represented major barriers to innovation and
- a continuous burden to people who were motivated to produce and implement innovative ideas.

3.7 Why Did the Innovation Fail

The lessons from this innovation which failed to be adopted are multiple. The key learning points are the following:

- The implementation of innovation including stakeholder engagement is the critical step in the innovation process which needs to be planned early and led well, at the stage of idea generation. The implementation plan should be robust enough to support early innovation adoption and subsequent diffusion and should include a well thought stakeholder engagement plan. Innovation in healthcare has multiple benefits associated with its implementation, financial and non-financial and those need to be well-defined. A clear evaluation strategy of the innovation implementation needs to be built into the implementation plan in order to evaluate the innovation benefits. The evaluation needs to start early on in the innovation process in order to capture the effectiveness of the preparation and engagement phase. This case illustrates a good example of an evaluation strategy but there was no robust implementation plan beyond the adoption phase. The implementation plan should have included a clear engagement strategy plan to enable not just the adoption but also the diffusion of innovation. The clinical innovator could have led a stakeholder mapping exercise to ensure that all stakeholders were considered and engaged appropriately and throughout the stages of innovation.

- Innovation adoption is the first step in the innovation journey, a prerequisite to innovation diffusion and requires strong clinical leader engagement. The role of the clinical innovator is key for ensuring there is enough critical mass of people (followers) who support the innovation. Having such critical mass enhances the chances of the innovation moving beyond the adoption stage. The lack of a wider oncology and healthcare system stakeholder commitment made the case for adoption of the innovation less compelling to the funding panel. The innovator could have engaged with innovators external to the organization who may have succeeded in getting similar innovations adopted and diffused in order to inspire and engage the clinical and non-clinical communities.
- It is not enough for an innovation to reach the pilot phase, because without an organized implementation plan (funds, people, capability, partners), the innovation is unlikely to move beyond the pilot phase. A short-term implementation pilot should have been supplemented by a long-term sustainable plan to diffuse

the innovation and scale it up in other clinical specialties and partnered organizations across the system. An early engagement of the local clinical commissioning group (CCG) and other system partners could have exposed the innovation to a wider supportive network. It could have led to other sources of funding in case the Innovate UK grant was unsuccessful. In addition, the financial risk could have been shared between Innovate UK and the clinical commissioning group in a more collaborative approach. Such a gesture could have given the confidence to the Innovate UK committee of the innovation's sustainability, which could have led to winning the grant.

- The identification and engagement of early adopters is key, including commissioners and providers. A comprehensive stakeholder engagement strategy at an organizational and system level needs to complement the entrepreneurial approach of local innovators (Martin et al. 2012; Hunter et al. 2012; Barker et al. 2016). This includes the selection and engagement of business partners. In this case, a combination of international and local enterprises were selected to work on the innovation. It is important that due diligence is done to support the choice of business partners. A lack of commitment and trust can be detrimental to the innovation adoption and diffusion.
- The application of the business modelling approach to innovation by Van Limburg et al. (2011), through the presentation of a clear and structured strategy for the evaluation of innovation was positively perceived by the innovation fund panel. However, the evaluation was not supplemented by a comprehensive stakeholder engagement strategy and the innovation run the risk of not been supported by commissioners in the long run and after the funded pilot ended. In that scenario, the

organization would have to bear the costs of continuing with the innovation which would have been financially unsustainable.

- The implementation and diffusion of innovations can be financially complex, especially when they involve collaborations between different organizations. There is a requirement for good commercial capabilities from the part of the leading organization (Williams et al. 2008). The innovation collaborative between the NHS, industry and academia, needed a better clarification and agreement of shared risks and rewards. In this case, even if the innovation fund had been awarded, the handling and distribution of funds across the lifetime of the project was a risk. The power dynamics between the three large stakeholders (NHS, industry, academia) were challenging and conversations around ownership of the innovation were not effective. As a result, there were issues around trust, commitment and integrity amongst the stakeholders regarding the innovation implementation timeline and the future beyond the funded pilot.

- Early executive engagement and commitment in the innovation process is key to innovation success. The organization's commitment to innovation should have gone beyond a top-down decision to adopt innovation through the Ideas Den. Endorsement of the innovation should have been accompanied by the necessary resources to support the implementation of the innovation beyond the pilot. This would have helped with the change management process, with clinician incentivisation and with the innovation team confidence on the value of the process. A quote from a senior member of the innovation team at the very start of the process, regarding the Ideas Den purpose and the Trust obligations, was the following:

> There will be an expectation for resource to make it happen, or mandate to work with an external company if our ICT department cannot support
>
> **NHS Transformation Manager**

- Early and continuous involvement of patients and the public is key in the adoption and diffusion of innovations in healthcare. In this scenario, there was good engagement of patients and the public who expressed their views on the innovation and its benefits. It is important that healthcare innovations with multiple benefits for patients and staff are supported by a robust implementation and scale up plan to ensure they are sustained beyond adoption. It would be unethical in this case to withdraw the innovation following the end of the pilot due to the lack of sustainable resources to support it. This was also a concern expressed by the innovation committee.
- Consideration needs to be given to prevent widening the gap of health inequalities in terms of access to healthcare. Digitising healthcare services bears the risk of depriving access to care for patients who are less technological savvy or they can't afford the wifi or other digital devices. A comprehensive innovation strategy should incorporate a population health component within its benefit realisation.
- Healthcare innovation adoption and diffusion is more likely to happen in the context of an autonomous and empowered workforce. The top-down control of the innovation process in this case meant that that the innovator's internal motivation to experiment and change model of care was not met with the respective support from the organization. It is documented that a centralized approach to innovation decision-making can stifle creativity and innovation (Damanpour and Schneider 2006).

3.8 Organizational Response to Innovation Failure

The digital innovation case demonstrated the need for fundamental leadership ingredients so that healthcare organizations succeed in innovation, such as an autonomous innovation department, innovators incentivization, co creation and innovator peer support, the presence of a viable innovation strategy that aligns with organizational vision, key end user and stakeholder engagement.

Following the innovation bid rejection, there was some reorganization within the Trust, with the majority of the innovation and transformation teams leaving the Trust including the project manager of the innovation project. The Innovation department started to collaborate much more closely with the Research & Development department and a business partner was appointed on a permanent basis to advice on intellectual property issues.

In addition, a new clinical lead for innovation was appointed to provide strong clinical leadership and engage more constructively with clinicians during their innovation journey. The clinical lead had strong partnerships with local universities, led a surgical research fellow program within the Trust and worked closely with industry partners which helped in getting industry support for innovation. A new Research and Development lead was also appointed who also had a professorial position in the local university and was well respected in the local community and nationally.

These organizational changes gave a positive signal to clinicians and potential innovators who continued to come forward with their ideas. The organization started to attract industry partners who engaged with the Trust seeking possible collaborations.

Although the innovation project did not receive the funding award and did not progress, the Trust reflected on the barriers to this innovation and others going on at the same time from succeeding and made positive steps forward to restructure the innovation and transformation teams. The constructive feedback offered by staff who were involved in the innovation project as well as the feedback from the external innovation funding committee, helped the Trust make the necessary changes to raise its innovation profile and consequently, raise the overall reputation of the organization. A new innovation and research strategy was written and supported by the newly appointed Innovation, Research and Development leads.

Innovation in the NHS is often initiated by front line clinicians (Harris and Bhatti 2016) who are highly self-motivated and is important that they operate in an environment that nurtures their competencies and autonomy to innovate (Ryan and Deci 2000). Such environments are more likely to stimulate clinician internal motivation and innovations are more likely to take off (Ryan and Deci 2000).

The failed digital innovation gave the impetus to change the way the Trust viewed Innovation and put the necessary resources to boost innovation in the years to come. The joined innovation and research strategy which was put forward had short, medium and long-term performance targets with the vision for the NHS Trust to become the leading UK organization when it comes to research and innovation. The joined innovation and research strategy was linked with the Trust's human resource and recruitment strategy to support the recruitment and retention of highly talented clinicians and innovators.

Bottom-up innovations need appropriate infrastructure, top-down support and strategic partnerships if they are to be adopted, diffused and sustained (Williams 2016). Shortage of those organizational capabilities may lead to innovations failing to become adopted and implemented. Innovation can be viewed as a change process within organizations and communication of a shared clear vision for innovation is key.

Involvement of end users early in the innovation process and ensuring co-creation of innovation with end users may also lead more often to the desired change (Al-Haddad and Kotnour 2015). End user involvement in the design, implementation and evaluation of innovation is essential and often guides innovation teams about which aspects of innovation to measure in the evaluation process. End user involvement in the data analysis is crucial in making sense of the outcomes of the evaluation as well as in the dissemination of the outcomes to the wider community.

References

Al-Haddad S, Kotnour T (2015) Integrating the organizational change literature: a model of successful change. J Organ Chang Manag 28(2):234–262

Barker PM, Reid A, Schall MW (2016) A framework for scaling up health interventions: lessons from large-scale improvement initiatives in Africa. Implement Sci 11:12

Barnett J, Vasileiou K, Fayika D et al (2011) Understanding innovators' experience of barriers and facilitators in implementation and diffusion of healthcare service innovations: a qualitative study. BMC Health Serv Res 11(342)

Basch E, Deal AM, Dueck AC et al (2017) Overall survival results of a trial assessing patient-reported outcomes for symptom monitoring during routine cancer treatment. JAMA

Chesbrough H, Bogers M (2014) Explicating open innovation: clarifying an emerging paradigm for understanding innovation. In: Chesbrough H, Vanhaverbeke W, West J (eds) New frontiers in open innovation. Oxford University Press, Oxford, pp 3–28

Damanpour F, Schneider M (2006) Phases of the adoption of innovation in organizations: effects of the environment, organization and top managers. Br J Manag 17:215–236

Dillon A, Morris M (1996) User acceptance of new information technology: theories and models. Ann Rev Inf Sci Technol 14(4):3–32

Etzkowitz H (2013) Innovation in innovation: the triple helix of university-industry-government relations. Soc Sci Inf 42(3):293–337

Ferlie E, Fitzgerald L, Wood M, Hawkins C (2005) Acad Manag J 48(1):117–134

Fukofuka S, Lokke DT (2015) OCTAPACE and organisational resilience: a correlational study. OJBMR 4(1):1–10

Greenhalgh T, Wherton J, Papoutsi C et al (2018) Analysing the role of complexity in explaining the fortunes of technology programmes: empirical application of the NASSS framework. BMC Med 16:66

Greenhalgh T (2018) How to improve success of technology projects in health and social care. Public Health Res Pract 28(3)

Griffiths F, Bryce C, Cave J et al (2017) Timely digital patient-clinician communication in specialist clinical services for young people: a mixed- methods study (the LYNC study). J Med Internet Res 19(4):e102

Harris M, Bhatti Y (2016) The global diffusion of healthcare innovation: making the connections. World Innov Summit Health

Hunter ST, Cushenbery L, Friedrich T (2012) Hiring an Innovative workforce: a necessary yet uniquely challenging endeavor. Hum Resour Manag Rev 22:303–322

Lundvall BA (2016) Product innovation and user-producer interaction in the learning economy and the economics of hope. Anthem Press, London, p 2016

Martin GP, Weaver S, Currie G et al (2012) Innovation sustainability in challenging health-care contexts. Health Serv Manag Res 25:190–199

Martinez-Cardoso D (2014) Taylor's scientific management principles in current organizational management practices. Organiz Behav Leadersh s141180

Money AG, Barnett J, Kuljis J et al (2011) The role of the user within the medical device design and development process: medical device manufacturers' perspectives. BMC Med Inform Decis Mak 11:15

Newman SP, Bardsley M, Barlow J et al (2011) Whole systems demonstrator programme

Nilsen ER, Dugstad J, Eide H et al (2016) Exploring resistance to implementation of welfare technology in municipal healthcare services—A longitudinal case study. BMC Health Serv Res 16:657

Omachonu VK, Einspruch NG (2010) Innovation in healthcare delivery systems: a conceptual framework. Innov J 15(1)

Rogers EM (1995) Diffusion of innovations, 4th edn. Free Press, New York

Ryan RM, Deci EL (2000) Self-determination theory and the facilitation of intrinsic motivation, social development and wellbeing. Am Psychol 55(1):68–78

Shah SGS, Robinson I (2007) Benefits of and Barriers to involving users in medical device technology development and evaluation. Int J Technol Assess Healthc 23(1):131–137

Van Limburg M, van Gemert-Pijnen J, Seydel ER (2011) Why business modelling is crucial in the development of eHealth Technologies. J Med Internet Res 13(4):e124

Vincent C, Blandford A (2011) Designing for safety and usability: user-centered techniques in medical device design practice. In: Proceedings of the human factors and ergonomics society annual meeting sage publications

Williams R (2016) Why is it difficult to achieve e-health systems at scale? Inf Commun Soc 19(4):540–550

Williams DJ, Wells O, Hourd P, Chandra A (2008) Feeling the pain: disruptive innovation in healthcare markets. Innov Manuf Netw

Winslow R (2016). New studies rely on the internet for help treating cancer patients [Blog]. Wall Street J

4

Learning from Innovation Success—*A Case Study*

Abstract In the private health sector, innovation happens because of the need to continually improve services or due to the need for differentiation and disruption, through the delivery of new product and services or expanding to new markets (Bolwijn and Kumpe 1990). The competitiveness of the external environment including the reduced barrier to entry and reimbursement challenges, makes innovation a necessity for the financial sustainability of private organizations. The private healthcare organization under study is young and entrepreneurial with the vision to expand its services and products to other markets, hence becoming the global provider of choice for cancer care. The innovation model adopted to expand its service offerings globally is cyclical and involves a number of innovations which are implemented at the same time, with one innovation driving the other (Berkhout et al. 2006). This model suits the organizational culture and vision, which includes the creation of multiple differentiators for the purpose of developing a unique service proposition for its customers (Berkhout et al. 2006). The strong organizational vision together with the entrepreneurial and risky organizational behaviour, align well with the cyclical innovation model (Bessant and Tidd 2013). The success of one innovation can be very influential and often one successful innovation can drive more innovation. This is a social innovation model which is characterised by a strong sense of organizational vision, a risky organizational behaviour and one that values partnerships within and between organizations (Bessant and Tidd 2013). The internal environment of the private organization differs to the NHS organization described in the previous section, in that it embraces risk and change, but is also more agile in its decision-making process for bringing innovative ideas to implementation. On the contrary, the NHS organization is more bureaucratic in its decision making and risk-averse when it comes to innovation and change. In the next few sections, the innovation journey of the private organization will be evaluated in terms of leadership strengths, enablers and barriers.

4.1 The Innovation Purpose

The studied innovation model is characterized by multiple innovations which serve the company mission pillars—*Quality*, *Access* and *Efficiency*. The model was applied for the purpose of transforming the company's breast cancer service across the whole patient pathway, from diagnosis through to treatment and survivorship.

The transformation process was triggered mainly by external forces, including:

- Competition with other private providers
- Competition with the single most powerful competitor—the NHS
- New entries to industry competing for same clinical workforce
- Technological advances in cancer diagnostics and radiotherapy treatments
- Year on year poor growth in patient referrals for treatment
- UK having the lowest survival in breast cancer compared to other European countries, with cancer waiting times standards often not being met (Papanicolas et al. 2019)
- Wide variation in the access and quality of breast radiotherapy in UK with poor progress in clinical protocol development and innovation (Livi et al. 2015).

All the above triggers led the company to create new and innovative services and blueprinting them through the breast cancer service transformation program. The program represented a whole system approach to change, involving a number of innovations across the whole patient pathway, from diagnosis through to survivorship. Innovations ranged from purely technical ones to service ones and also digital innovations. The learnings and the 'know-how' from the breast cancer transformation program would be used to transform other clinical services within the organization and the group as a whole. This was an opportunity for the company to make a real difference to patient outcomes and improve its reputation.

The diffusion of innovations within a network of private centres was optimised using a whole systems approach to change. This approach started with the top-down creation of the vision for change, the description and measurement of future desired outcomes, followed by stakeholder engagement internally and externally (Blizzard and Klotz 2012; Crompton-Phillips 2020). On the contrary, there was no shared vision amongst stakeholders in the NHS digital innovation case and there were important stakeholders that were not engaged, such as doctors, commissioners and integrated care practitioners such as GPs. We believe that the bottom-up only approach to the digital innovation process in the NHS, without the top-down leadership and support did not result in the adoption of the innovation. The private organization utilised the principles of the tight-loose-tight model by Crompton-Phillips (2020), ensuring there was a right balance between setting the direction for change (top-down) and allowing front line leaders to lead the implementation of individual innovations (bottom-up). The combination of bottom-up innovation implementation and top-down leadership support can ensure that front line staff have a sense of autonomy and freedom to experiment whilst feeling supported in taking risks when innovating (Fukofuka and Lokke 2015).

The breast cancer service innovation program involved a top-down strategy at first, unlike the digital innovation in the NHS which was driven solely by a front-line clinical innovator with no decision-making powers. In this case, the sponsor of the innovation program was an executive member of the UK leadership team (medical director) and the creator of the program (the innovator). The innovator had the decision-making power to drive strategy top-down as well as the clinical knowledge to support the strategy bottom-up. The high-level strategy was shared with all the UK centre managers and front-line staff but without much involvement of them in co-creating the innovation strategy. The expectation was that middle managers and front-line leaders, as well as clinical leaders, would be heavily involved in the implementation of the strategy through the different innovation workstreams, which is where they would have the opportunity to shape and influence the innovation process.

Obtaining internal support and buy-in on the strategy was helpful in the creation of a shared internal organizational vision and purpose. The internal people engagement piece ensured that the innovation strategy was well supported by the whole organization. By doing so, the organization could maximize the external engagement piece, targeting the main end users, patients and doctors (referrers to the service).

End users such as consultant doctors and patients were not consulted in the proposal early on, because of the urgency of producing a plausible strategy ahead of other competitors. Revealing the strategy too early meant that they would be introducing an unnecessary risk of the strategy being replicated by other providers, gaining competitive advantage and competing for the same clientele (doctors referring to their service). The doctors and referrers were not employees of the organization, which meant that there needed to be a strategic approach to clinical engagement and a requirement to keep the strategy confidential until an implementation plan was formulated and under way (Shah and Robinson 2007).

The forecasted financial benefits from the strategy implementation were significant which also led to the swift implementation of the strategy before an extensive engagement piece with end users. The opportunity to improve patient outcomes by introducing service innovations was a plausible strategy, as there was enough clinical evidence behind the proposed innovations. The specialized technological nature of the innovation portfolio meant that patients would not be in a position to be involved in the co-creation of the innovation strategy. Patient engagement in the form of patient experience forums came at a later stage in the innovation process and particularly during the implementation and diffusion stage rather than the initial knowledge creation and adoption stages.

Primary and secondary care clinicians (GPs, Oncologists, Surgeons) were the main stakeholders to take on board during the adoption stage of the innovation process. Although the tactic of late end user involvement in the innovation process deprived the innovation team of a broad clinical and patient intelligence in the creation of innovation, at the same time it eliminated the risk of the innovation program being resisted by end users. The innovation process involved significant internal cultural change in the way care was delivered by the organization. There was also a significant digital transformation component which would enable more efficient and safer clinical workflows. The focus was therefore given to ensuring that the internal workforce was engaged well at the start of the process as everyone within the company would then work together to engage the external stakeholders. Executive managers and commissioners of the innovation program had complete buy-in because of the expected improvement in care outcomes and also the forecasted significant revenue to the business (Money et al. 2011).

The organization applied a nationally approved change management model in order to transform its breast cancer service offering. The change management model followed quality improvement principles: the implementation of the six steps to quality improvement change (Jones et al. 2019). Utilising a whole system approach to change, the innovation process began with vision creation, scope building and outcome definition, led by the medical director (Blizzard and Klotz 2012). This was followed by a series of presentations to the wider organization and various engagement events with all staff members (front line to executives) on a national, but also a global scale where the company operated. What followed the engagement events was an internal recruitment strategy for subject matter experts (SMEs) who would form workstreams to implement the innovations. In addition, there was a detailed operational strategy formed to enable all UK centres get ready for the implementation and diffusion stage of the innovation process. Finally, there was an intense education and engagement program during the adoption stage and devoted to clinical end users, including oncologists, surgeons and GPs, but also internal staff. This educational program also aimed at identifying innovation champions (subject matter experts) who would work with the organization workforce in the piloting, evaluation, refinement, diffusion and scaling up of innovations (Jones et al. 2019).

The types of innovations included in the program involved technological enhancements, new digital tools, research and development services, whole service transformation methods and external partnerships. Based on the whole system change theory, the program was planned robustly in terms of scoping and strategizing, shared vision formulation, financial and non-financial benefit realization planning and an evaluation process was embedded in the program. Monitoring of program milestones was performed by the executive program board led by the medical director (the innovator and sponsor of innovation) and other members of the UK leadership team. The executive program board was supportive of the internal workforce taking part in workstream activities and some staff members were also seconded to new roles to support the innovation program. The fact that the UK leadership team created the safe space as well as new roles to support the innovation program, motivated front-line staff to pursue innovation as business-as-usual.

Internal and external stakeholder workshops supplemented the formal executive board meetings and informed the board of any refinements needed to the innovations through the workstream leads. Clinical staff with various positions within the organization, including doctors (end users), nurses, radiographers, physicists, pharmacists and healthcare assistants participated in the workshops which had an engaging, learning and knowledge disseminating nature (Glew 2002). Feedback from those meetings was used to refine innovation implementation, ensuring robust implementation and future innovation sustainability. Patients did not participate in the workshops but were informed of the progress of various innovations through newsletters and patient experience workshops (end user testing of innovations). Patients were not present in the project board either, but they were represented by a dedicated patient experience lead who also facilitated the patient experience workshops. Internal and external stakeholder engagement and feedback were all part of the innovation process. The participatory nature of the innovation process made it more likely for staff to become engaged and the programme to lead to positive outcomes quickly and within one year of strategy conception.

The organisation took the risk to change the status quo in breast cancer care, whilst learning from experimentation (de Ven 2017). The breast program innovations were executed by exploiting existing resources and networks and ensuring execution was replicated and scaled across the UK network. The innovation program in the private sector managed to exploit existing resources without a heavy investment in technologies and workforce, ensuring operational efficiencies. For example, front line clinical and non-clinical staff had their role extended and were incentivised to take on extra roles within the innovation process, by offering space in their working day to perform their new roles. There was also protected time for them to be internally trained on new skills to be able to perform new roles, which opened up future new permanent roles for them within the organization. Some staff were offered a secondment role to support with specialised areas of interest to them such as IT, digital, research and data analytics and some people moved permanently into innovation positions to support specialised interest roles. Other exploitation strategies included the expansion of an existing virtual platform to perform remote multidisciplinary consultations, the creation of an internal breast cancer clinical reference group (CRG) from existing doctor (referrer) pool who championed the innovations and the use of the existing electronic health record to record patient reported outcomes. In the NHS digital innovation case, the Trust did not exploit its existing IT business partnerships, workforce capacity and existing electronic health record to drive innovation. We believe that this represented a missed opportunity for innovation for the NHS Trust.

4.2 Leadership Enablers and Barriers to Innovation

The breast cancer innovation program was ambitious with 24 innovations in the process of implementation within a 12-month timeline target. The '*Access*' component of the innovation program was the most successful; it mostly involved the clinical-technical radiotherapy service innovations which were adopted and diffused across the network within 12 months.

The diffusion success of those innovations can be attributed mainly to the intense education program for clinicians which the organization delivered early on during the adoption phase

Head of Radiotherapy Services

The educational strategy which was led by the innovator, a senior clinician and medical director in the organization, required considerable clinician training and behaviour modelling. The steps taken by the innovator with support from the organization in order to change clinician behaviour and promote the adoption and diffusion of innovative radiotherapy techniques are as follows:

- Presentations of the clinical evidence to clinicians (active, in-person strategy), through the delivery of key opinion leader workshops;
- Distribution of an innovation journal to clinicians including all quantitative evidence of patient benefit from those techniques;
- Clinician credentialing program through a targeted educational strategy;
- Establishment of a peer review process for radiotherapy planning;
- The offering of a 24/7 technical support for clinicians during planning;
- Clinician engagement in the deployment of an auto-contouring radiotherapy tool;
- Creation of a virtual cancer multidisciplinary forum for case discussion;
- Utilization of Clinician champions of the innovations through the creation of a breast clinical reference group;
- Engagement of an international key opinion leader as an advocate of the innovations to the UK oncological community;

- Internal recruitment of a trained advanced practitioner, expert in advanced breast radiotherapy planning to support clinicians during their radiotherapy planning.

The above tactical steps aimed at maximising innovation implementation and diffusion, compared to simple dissemination of clinical evidence. Those steps enabled the achievement of the desired outcome for the 'Access' component of the innovation program which were all implemented and diffused within 12 months.

> The breast cancer strategy for Access has improved the quality of radiotherapy techniques and made it more personalised to patient needs
>
> **Radiographer 1**

The challenges that the leadership team faced during the adoption and diffusion of the technical innovations were mainly due to the mixed opinions amongst clinicians regarding the usefulness of the innovations. Despite the fact that there was clear clinical evidence suggestive of the beneficial role of such innovative techniques over standard techniques, most clinicians were initially not convinced that a change in practice was worth it at the time. The existing evidence was also interpreted differently amongst clinicians, leading to a non-uniform endorsement of the techniques and limited to a minority of clinical innovation champions. This hindered the initial adoption and spread of the innovations across the network. One of the most successful tactical strategies was the involvement of the international key opinion leader who led on the educational sessions for the UK clinician network.

> The move to bring over to UK the single doctor who has revolutionised breast radiotherapy globally was smart and the right thing to do
>
> **Consultant Oncologist 1**

The role of clinical leadership through the innovator, the few clinician champions and the international key opinion leader, was critical for the ongoing education, encouragement and clinician support in the adoption and diffusion of those innovations. They acted as knowledge brokers (Sousa 2008; Cillo 2005) by bringing external knowledge and linking this knowledge with the internal innovation capabilities of the organization. An open innovation approach was followed with clinicians from different practices and centres collaborating for the creation of new protocols and workflows to improve the breast cancer service proposition (Sousa 2008). The extensive experience of those leaders and the sharing of such knowledge in the form of educational events with regular knowledge reinforcement, resulted in the increase in patient referrals for those techniques. The peak of referrals coincided with the timing of the educational sessions. Those sessions not only gave clinicians the opportunity to enhance their knowledge and skills but also enabled them to network with their peers on a regular basis. The sessions also brought clinicians closer to the organization management team and improved their trusting relationship with the company.

Other challenges to the radiotherapy innovation adoption and diffusion and the ways those were addressed through leadership, were as follows:

- *The lack of robust and pre-existing clinician training in radiotherapy planning using those innovative techniques*: this was addressed through knowledge brokers, clinical championship and information transferring via means of educational events and workshops. The technical innovation training enhanced clinician specialised skills, led to knowledge spread across the national oncology network, increased the interaction with international key opinion leaders and ultimately increased the confidence of clinicians to adopt innovation in oncology.

- *The lack of clinician incentivisation in terms of available time spent planning compared to more standard and less complex radiotherapy techniques*: addressed through the provision of an advanced radiotherapy practitioner, 24 h IT support and through the deployment of an auto-contouring software tool.
- *The lack of a peer support process for clinicians to gain confidence in advanced radiotherapy planning*: this was addressed through the provision of internal digital and technological tools to enable clinicians to peer review their radiotherapy plans with other colleagues.
- *Clinician remuneration was not higher to compensate for the technique complexity and clinician time consumed to deliver the techniques*. The organization managed the resistance from clinicians to adopt the new techniques through the provision of advanced planning support and the deployment of an auto-contouring radiotherapy tool which reduced clinician time to plan.
- *The lack of a cohesive, early adopter breast group to guide on protocols and guidelines* was mitigated through the creation of a breast clinical reference group consisting of innovation champions. They led the adoption of new guidelines and clinical protocols, peer reviewed from international experts in the field.

It became clear that turning challenges into enablers required strong leadership, clinical and managerial leadership. The medical director and members of the executive leadership team used tactics such as smart investment in AI-trained tool to improve process efficiencies, the use of existing digital platforms and own workforce in order to support process and drive clinicians to adopt practice change.

The catalyst to changing clinician behaviour leading to the adoption and diffusion of the radiotherapy techniques, was the targeted educational strategy that was designed by the innovator. There were three workshops strategically planned to happen every few months to ensure regular clinician knowledge reinforcement.

> The workshops gave the opportunity to clinicians nationally to credential themselves through being taught by an international expert who teaches and credentials oncologists around the world
> **Operational Middle Manager**

The educational workshops were designed by clinicians for clinicians and there was less top-down power in those sessions. The power was redirected from top-down to bottom-up, and clinicians felt in control of the clinician networking and credentialing process. They also felt empowered and valued by the organization, as the management team listened and addressed their concerns which were putting barriers to the adoption of those techniques (incentivisation, upskilling, supportive planning team, peer review digital tool, IT support).

> The creation of an endorsing community of clinicians was important as any perceived risk was shared amongst a body of professionals
> **Business development manager 1**

The perceived increased workload by clinicians was one significant barrier to the adoption and diffusion of the techniques, similar to the NHS innovation case.

The perception of workload demands careful consideration when healthcare organizations look to implement innovations.

The organizational leadership team addressed clinician concerns by investing in the training of advanced practitioners internally to support clinicians during planning and by investing in a radiotherapy planning tool that enabled auto-contouring through the use of machine-learning technology. The company's response to clinician resistance demonstrates the importance of an entrepreneurial organizational culture and a risk-taking behaviour from its leaders when it comes to innovation. Such organizational response was not evident in the digital innovation case in the NHS which resulted in the innovation idea stalling. The company's response was also key in bridging the gap between the top-down strategic approach and front-line clinical leader involvement.

The risk of not responding to the clinician resistance the way they did was the loss of clinician clientele and becoming worse-off financially.

Looking at the innovations around *'Quality'* and *'Efficiency'*, there are some distinct differences in the degree of diffusion amongst them. For example, innovations were implemented and diffused early if significant clinician involvement was required. Clinicians were mostly motivated to implement those for reputational, professional (clinical benefit to patients) and financial benefits. Those successful innovations included:

- The establishment of *One Stop clinics* across the network, which provided easy access for patients to be seen by a specialist on demand, have a full work-up of tests and receive rapid diagnosis;
- The *e-referral and referrer support process* which enabled general practitioners, patients (self-referrals), surgeons and other clinicians from across the UK to refer

patients to the One Stop clinics and other services, quickly and accurately;
- The *virtual e-MDT* (cancer multidisciplinary team) tool which enabled the breast clinical reference group and others to meet up anytime there was a need to discuss patient cases or for treatment peer review purposes.

Those three innovative services were interdependent in the sense that one innovation brought the next and they were all hugely disruptive to the market. They led to the expansion of clinical services, the recruitment of an increasing number of doctors as a result, which in turn brought a higher number of patient referrals and greater reputation for the organisation. Clinicians were in full control of the service innovation developments and the business utilized its internal operational capabilities to the maximum in order to support the quick implementation of those services, within 12 months from the strategy conception.

In contrast, the adoption of other innovations which did not require clinicians, they did not confer immediate benefits to patients and clinicians and were mostly management-led, did not take off as quickly. Those included patient registries and clinical research including clinical trials. The reasons behind this are multiple:

- Clinicians are risk-averse by nature and are motivated by quick-win results, therefore did not see a flourishing opportunity for them in the clinical trial and research development space;
- The delivery of clinical trial results can take considerable time and effort as well as research expertise, which the majority of clinicians lacked;
- Clinical trial delivery depends on a robust clinical trial governance infrastructure to oversee the implementation of trials. In turn this requires considerable

investment in a research and development workforce. In this organization, clinical trial delivery heavily relied upon the principal investigators which were the clinicians treating the patients. The time and cost associated with setting up a robust research and development team meant that clinicians had to give up sessions in their clinical practice in order to devote themselves to clinical trials. Although the organization was prepared to bear the cost and investment in research and clinical trials, clinicians were not prepared to compromise their high volume standard clinical practice.

- Patient registries did not take off as quickly and they were just beginning to be implemented by the end of the 12 months, following the creation of a digital registry tool. We believe that the main reason for the implementation delay was the need for dedicated clinician time to complete the digital registry tool, which was outside their standard of care provision.

One of the strategies used to encourage clinicians to lead on clinical trials including setting up and completing clinical registries, was the set-up of collaborations between the organization and research active teams based in nearby academic institutions. By the end of the study period (12 months), the senior leadership team had created some partnerships with two academic institutions in UK and started working on some collaborative clinical trials. Having the support of academic institutions in terms of clinical trial governance and leadership, the clinicians could then focus on recruiting patients which most were willing to do. In addition, the active encouragement by academics to have patient data systematically collected through patient registries, led to clinicians seeing the value of registries for analysing and improving patient outcomes.

> We need the universities to work with us on the registry and clinical trial front, to support us in trial applications but also ensure a robust governance process along the way
> **Commercial Director 1**

The lack of strong clinician incentivisation in terms of time and space to grow the clinical trial and registry portfolio, as well as the lack of immediate clinician rewards from such strategy, meant that clinical trials were not adopted during the time of the study. However, the senior medical leadership and executive team developed a favourable environment for clinicians to still be engaged in clinical trials through external partnerships. The collaborative environment between academics and clinical staff set the foundations for a growing research department within the organization, which was launched after the 12-month innovation programme period.

The creation of a patient portal system capability was part of the innovation strategy to improve quality and efficiency of communication between patients and their clinical teams. Although this was a top-down strategy, clinicians were involved in the choice to 'buy' the service or 'make' the service. The decision to create a bespoke system, which could be used by all three countries where the company operated, meant that the innovation could not be adopted and diffused at the time of study. The preliminary scoping exercise of what the system could look like and the definition of the global vision around this new model of care, was made collaboratively between the senior leaders of the three countries with clinician representation from the breast clinical reference group. The innovation was subsequently moved to a dedicated global team for implementation and moved away from the breast service transformation portfolio.

Exercise medicine and wellbeing services were implemented and diffused across the network pretty quickly, but they required a significant investment by the organization in terms of building gym facilities and hiring wellbeing consultants across the centres. The implementation of integrative oncology facilities such as exercise and wellbeing services was innovative and aligned with the purpose and values of the organization. Those innovations were highly valued by clinicians and patients alike due to the benefit that they brought in terms of improving patient outcomes, the reputation of the centres and attracting more patient referrals. Clinical leaders' role was mainly supportive and they were not heavily involved in the implementation of the innovations in their individual centres.

> This is a service 'nice to have' which will attract patient referrals and clinicians won't have to put any effort on it. Everyone loves that service
>
> **Centre leader 1**

Consequently, there was no resistance to those innovations by the vast majority of clinicians. There were very few clinicians who were concerned with their patients exercising during treatment. However, patient voice was so positive and strong around exercise and cancer, that even the most sceptical clinicians were eventually convinced. The purpose of the organization was to ensure best possible life outcomes for patients and such a movement gave the right message to clinicians and patients. The organization also gained through increasing its reputation as being the world's biggest integrative oncology provider which resulted in the onboarding of more clinicians. The introduction of such health and wellbeing facilities attracted more patients who wanted to be treated in those facilities.

Finally, the pursue of an integrative medicine approach led to strategic partnerships which helped raise the profile of the organisation at a global scale.

Other innovations like patient reported outcome measures (PROMs) and genomic testing were adopted but variably diffused across the network.

- The idea around PROMs was that they would be collected during treatment and post treatment from patients and facilitated through an App which patients would have access to. The collection and evaluation of PROMs could help evaluate and refine aspects of service. It would also support future research and quality improvement initiatives.
- Genomic testing for patients enables clinicians to individualise patient treatments and know the risk of cancer recurrence for their patients. This involves testing an existing tumour sample, doing a blood test or both and checking for specific mutations in the tumour which could guide clinician treatment decision-making.

Both innovations needed to be clinically driven due to their specialised nature. Clinical leadership heavily influenced the implementation of those innovation, but different doctor leaders advocated for different PROMs and genomic test tools. A significant proportion of doctors felt that those innovations were not important elements in the overall breast cancer service quality. The availability of genomic testing and patient reported outcome measures did not have a direct impact on patient treatment and were therefore not viewed as immediate priorities for clinicians. Other factors contributing to the resistance to consider the adoption of genomic testing were the multitude of genomic tests in the market, combined with the immature knowledge of clinicians around genomic testing.

There are so many tests to choose from and frankly, it is very confusing for us all

Chemotherapy nurse 1

There were also no clear guidelines of when and how to use them and the process of requesting and reporting the tests required some effort from clinicians. Moreover, testing would delay patient treatment slightly which often made clinicians uncomfortable. Finally, the genomic service was thought to be a highly specialised area which required significant clinical control into the decision-making. The company was ambitious to make a change and a breakthrough into the genomic space, through engaging with key business partners and attempting to arrange an educational conference around genomics. Clinicians did not share the same vision though and were not ready for such change, especially in such a debatable and ethically challenging subject as genomics.

Few clinicians were individually approached by testing companies who engaged them well. It therefore became difficult to direct clinicians towards one test over another. It was therefore left to clinicians to make the choice of the right test for the right patient, often in consultation with their colleagues, breast clinical reference group and in the context of multi-disciplinary meetings. It is likely that the genomic testing service will mature in the future and become more uniformly diffused, as clinicians grow in confidence and trust on the use genomics in personalising care.

The case for change around PROMs was not met with resistance given the clear benefit for patients. However, there were similar issues as with genomic testing, in terms of the lack of national and international guidelines and no agreed process on how to collect and analyse them. In addition, the process needed clinician oversight and a clear patient engagement plan by clinicians to ensure patient reporting compliance. The organization attempted to standardize PROM collection through the involvement of a global clinical leader forum who agreed on standard PROMs to collect. In addition, the UK company invested on an App for patients to access and report their outcomes remotely. Not all clinicians were in favour of that approach, but an initial pilot showed that at least 50% of patients were compliant in their PROM reporting, a result which made clinicians feel more encouraged and motivated about it. The alternative solution which was also piloted was a PROM survey at the time when patient attended the centre or through a facilitated phone-call. Although this option ensured near 100% patient compliance, it was time consuming for centre staff. At the end, both options were adopted depending on the centre, clinician and patient preference. However, data quality was variable which led to the company decision to incorporate PROM collection and analysis into the future patient portal.

Finally, the cardio-Oncology service did not take off as a new service unlike the One stop Breast clinics. Some suggested reasons from various stakeholders were the following:

> The cardio-Oncology service involved the introduction of a new clinical specialty in the organization, which was outside the UK expertise
> **Service development manager**

> The cardio-Oncology service was considered by doctors as a non-essential service to have in-house and one that could be outsourced if and when required
> **Head of diagnostics**

Cardio-Oncology is not much developed as a specialty in the NHS practice and managers are not very familiar with operationalising such service, unlike the One stop diagnostic service
Consultant Oncologist and Clinical Director 2

We want to do a pilot in our centre but the investment on the service exceeds the financial returns
Centre leader 2

Maybe we need to outsource the service if and when required rather than providing the service in-house
Head of diagnostics

4.3 Perception of the Innovation Process and Leadership by Stakeholders

The overall perception of the innovation process by the various stakeholders was that the organization was very ambitious in trying to implement 24 innovations in 12 months. The vision was to adopt and diffuse all of the innovations in 12 months, creating a unique service proposition, which was more like a 2–3-year transformation plan.

Stakeholders who were involved in the innovation process described the process as cyclical and dynamic; the model enabled the diffusion of innovations at different times. Couple of innovations were temporarily dropped with the plan to be re-introduced at a later stage, as in the case of the patient portal. Cyclical innovation models or 4th generation models like the one described in this case involve whole systems, include product and service innovations, are flexible and agile, and reflect the organizational creativity and entrepreneurship. They also respond to the ever-changing demands of the competitive market, scientific knowledge and societal demands (Van Der Duin et al. 2007; Berkhout et al. 2006).

> The innovation model is uniquely disruptive, taking the breast cancer offering into a different dimension
>
> **CEO**

> The company is leading the way globally in terms of breast cancer innovations
>
> **Medical Director non-UK Business**

The innovation model became a company strategy, with plans to complete this cycle of innovation and start another in a year's time (version 2). Stakeholders involved in the innovation process bought into this model which became something like a blueprint for innovation execution, with plans to scale the program in other countries and other cancer specialties.

> Innovations which succeeded in being diffused would be dropped after the 12-month period and others would be introduced, in a continuous cycle of innovation
>
> **Business development manager 2**

The innovation process would become a continuous journey of improvement for the organization in the years to come. Succeeding in at least half of the innovations in year 1 being diffused, represented a great success story and most stakeholders' opinion was that the process was partially successful after 12 months.

> The innovation program was at least 'partially-successful' but some innovations were not diffused within the timeline
>
> **Commercial director 2**

In terms of the leadership capability and leadership styles during the innovation process, there was a variety of views from the various stakeholders which will be explored in more detail in the next section.

> Leadership was mainly top-down and driven from a position of power
>
> **Consultant Oncologist 2**

The medical director supported by the UK leadership team defined the innovation strategy and its various components before presenting the strategy internally first and then externally. The vision for the innovation strategy aligned well with the company's vision and values, which resonated with internal staff, hence they bought into the strategy. However, the strategy was not co-created with the involvement of internal staff or external clinicians. What followed was an intense 12-month period where staff had to balance their day-to-day operational pressures with innovation implementation. The feedback received from people on the front line was that the pressure to deliver the strategy was intense, especially as they strongly believed in the vision and purpose of the program.

> The leadership style from senior management was directive and ambitious, focusing on the outcomes rather than the innovation journey itself
>
> **Physicist**

Such a directive approach from senior leaders was somewhat performance driven with the achievement of financial outcomes at the end of the year. This performance driven approach went against what clinicians valued most, which is making the process of innovation open, transparent and clinically driven, with focus on clinical outcomes (bottom-up leadership).

> The process of innovation involved more people in management positions who added little value to the delivery of the products and services
> **Business development manager 1**

> The management team should have stepped back and acted as the enablers for clinicians to run the innovation process themselves
> **Head of Radiotherapy**

Neither the clinicians nor the patients were included early enough, in the creation stage of the strategy. The consequence of this was that there were certain innovations that were met with resistance and failed to be universally diffused, such as genomic testing and PROMs. Clinicians were more likely to be involved in innovations which had direct benefit to their patients and to the growth of their practice. They also looked for innovations which are easy to implement, not time-consuming, there were national or international guidelines supporting their implementation and key opinion leader expertise they could draw from.

> Leadership during the program was tenacious and kept going with different tactics despite resistance to change from clinicians
> **Business development manager 2**

Keeping going enabled transformational change in the organization to happen quickly and efficiently. The articulation of a vision by the medical director (top-down) which was based on long-term business growth and improvement in patient care stimulated employees to engage in innovation and commit themselves to the long-term goals. The support from the executive and global teams also maximized the effects of the vision creation and program purpose which increased performance.

Leadership was considered to be key in achieving the required clinician behavioural change and leaders had a clear vision and strategy that resonated with all levels within the organization.

> Leaders established clear but ambitious goals and worked with the people to bring the required change
>
> **Dosimetrist**

Good leadership meant that there was honest recognition that the innovation process was imperfect; there were innovations which worked well and were likely to be sustained following some investment from the organization and others which wouldn't diffuse because perhaps the organization, the market or both were not ready for them. Some examples included the genomic testing strategy, patient registries and the private clinical trial strategy.

> Leaders were honest about the proposed innovations that needed to stop as they didn't fit with the culture of the organization, as in the case of the breast key workers
>
> **Senior nurse leader**

The proposed breast key worker service was never implemented in the way that was intended and this was probably the only innovation that did not reach adoption stage. Although the scheme is well established in the public sector, the private centre teams were small and completely immersed into patient journeys from diagnosis through to survivorship. There was therefore no need for separate key workers for patients. This proposal would have been removed from the innovation program if this was co-created with front-line staff.

Positive aspects of leadership in the innovation process include the quality and frequency of communication with all stakeholders, the continuous request from leaders for stakeholder input during implementation, the good dissemination of progress updates and the continuous education and improvement of innovations. In addition, there was a strong alignment between the commercial, marketing and referrer engagement teams and the innovation strategy which meant that product and service innovations moved quickly from the design to implementation to commercialization (Van Der Duin et al. 2007).

The strong entrepreneurial nature of the business meant that there was a risk-taking behaviour from the leadership of the organization who invested in workforce, IT and digital tools in order to gain the trust and confidence of the clinicians. The leadership team had a strong vision and stress tested the innovations with the market before devising the strategic direction. This led to company investing on the delivery of the innovations first, followed by clinician engagement and getting clinician buy-in subsequently. Without the top-down leadership, sensing the opportunity and valuing of the innovations as well as the changing needs of the society and the market, it is unlikely that the innovations would have been diffused as quickly as they did.

4.4 Deep Dive into Leadership at Different Innovation Stages

Jones et al. (2019) described the organizational improvement and innovation journey as a whole system approach to change. The prerequisite of a successful improvement journey is the senior leaders in the organization setting the vision and purpose which then translates into an organization-wide strategy. An inclusive, supportive and nurturing leadership style from top leaders is what is needed to keep the internal motivation of the people who will deliver the innovation agenda (Waldman and Bass 1991). Compassionate leadership which involves the inspiration for a long-term vision, the creation of an empowering culture of autonomy and safety to experiment and the promotion of distributed leadership for innovation are key leadership elements for innovation success (West et al. 2017).

The cyclical innovation process was set up by senior leaders in the organization whose vision was to make the organization the best integrated care provider globally when it comes to the breast cancer service proposition, drawing from excellence around the world. This vision which resonated with all grades within the organization was built up to become a defined and ambitious strategy which was designed top-down but subsequently became part of the day-to-day practice for all staff. Everyone in the organization, from the front-line clinical to middle management to executives had a leadership role during the implementation of the strategy. Distributed leadership was enacted mainly at the diffusion and implementation stage of the innovation. Some stakeholders were of the opinion that the innovation program was more directional from top-down management than it was driven from the bottom-up at its initial stages of ideation and adoption. However, the latter did not compromise the success of the innovation program. The top-down approach in setting the innovation program was supported by the medical director in the organization who took the link role between the creation of the breast innovation strategy and the implementation in clinical practice. The innovation strategy was completely aligned with the vision and mission of the organization and resonated well with internal staff.

Innovations are more likely to diffuse and be implemented if they are supported by the end users and in this case, the doctors who would refer patients for treatment in the organization (Currie and Spyridonidis 2018). They are also more likely to be diffused if they fit the context and the environment within which they will be implemented (Currie and Spyridonidis 2018). In this case, engagement of key opinion leaders (KOLs) from outside the UK healthcare systems who had succeeded in the diffusion of those innovations, was a brave and risky move due to the probable resistance from UK clinicians. The risk was the disengagement of the UK doctors who could have considered the innovations irrelevant to the UK practice. However, the opposite happened, UK doctors became very engaged in the process of change and took an active part in educational and training workshops and events. The bravery exhibited from the senior medical leader through bringing international expertise into the organization rather than leading the whole education and clinical change internally, demonstrated that distributed leadership is powerful and can cross organizational boundaries.

Distributed leadership in this case was represented well through the whole system approach to change (Jones et al. 2019) which was used to implement the strategy. Leadership was devolved to multiple people (clinical and managerial) who belonged to workstream groups and who led individual aspects of the strategy, rather than being the responsibility of a single heroic leader (Crevani et al. 2007).

Innovations were packaged well and there was something for everyone to work on. By doing so, there was more ownership amongst clinicians and managers on innovations, which increased motivation and got rid of siloed working.

The senior medical leader flexed the leadership style between command and control and a visionary and empowering style, according to the circumstances. The majority of stakeholders thought that a directional and tenacious leadership style was necessary in order for the project not to be derailed and for the senior medical leader to work with people's resistance. Harris (2008) in Hao et al. (2017) supports the flexible directive leadership style of the principal leader during innovation, in terms of playing the person accountable for innovation success and ensuring alignment of leaders with shared vision and goals when required.

The influence of international clinical leadership was welcomed by the organization staff including doctors, as there was no competition or power exerted between them and the UK clinicians, due to their leadership been practiced in different healthcare systems to the UK. Education and training engagement of doctors created the passion and the vision to bring clinical-technical innovations to practice, sooner than it would have normally taken them in the public sector to do. The social networking, the peer review support and the continuous knowledge reinforcement sessions which brought the doctor community together, worked in favour of the innovation process more so than the clinical evidence per se (Dopson et al. 2002). Clinical champions who showed passion, bravery and agency early on in the engagement events came together to form the breast clinical reference group who advised the company and led the multidisciplinary peer review meetings.

Some of the technical and digital innovations could have been diffused faster following adoption, with the identification of local key opinion leaders or clinical peers. Distributed clinical leadership at all levels introduced earlier on in the process, would have potentially engaged more clinicians earlier on in the innovation process (Dopson et al. 2002). The need for early and shared leadership amongst clinicians was even more critical in the UK business, because clinicians were not employees of the organization. As a result, there was no direct incentive for them to engage in the change process. In addition, the majority of the doctors had no devoted time to drive the engagement strategy and pursue the education of their peers. Early and targeted clinician engagement would have helped understand the 'what's in it for me' aspect and target those clinicians with specialist interests. By doing so, some innovations such as genomic testing and clinical trials may have reached the adoption stage earlier.

The role of the clinician peer opinion leader was played by the medical director, who was also practising in the breast cancer field like the others and was an early adopter of innovations, but with an added vested interest in promoting the innovations for the benefit of the organization and the wider group. With the support of the UK senior leadership team, the medical director led a number of roadshows whereby internal and external clinical teams, from local NHS hospitals were invited to engage in open conversation about the purpose of the innovations, the evidence behind them and the different product and service developments. The medical director played the role of the leader who initiated the innovation strategy and inspired people to follow, but also played the middle-agent and facilitator who bridged the gap between strategy and operational execution (Burgess and Currie 2013). The operational execution was led by the centre teams in collaboration with clinicians and the clinical reference group, who all took part in our or more workstreams. There was often a differential engagement response from clinicians based on what innovations were important to them, their existing clinical practice, vested interests and their organizational context (Dopson et al. 2002). Regular project communication updates and celebrations for achievements took place during the engagement events to keep clinicians and internal staff motivated.

The engagement of the internal workforce early on in the strategy formulation demonstrated the inclusive and nurturant leadership behaviour of the organization. The fact that people were given leadership roles at different innovation workstreams projected a sense of autonomy and trust to the people across the organization, some of whom were seconded or permanently moved to new positions of interest. The innovation vision and purpose created a swift change in the culture of the organization and united people for the purpose of the common goal (Jones et al. 2019).

The execution of the innovation strategy became the focus of the front line, middle managers and senior leaders and was aligned with the commercial and marketing strategy which helped the dissemination of innovation products and services as they were launched. By the end of year 1, the breast service transformation strategy had led the foundations of an organizational culture where innovation was part of the day-to-day business and not a one-off activity (Millar et al. 2018). This was achieved through shared leadership and ownership of innovation diffusion within the organization, for the purpose of changing care models to improve patient outcomes.

End user (doctor) involvement did not take place early on during the strategy formulation and innovation conception stage, instead the agenda for innovation in the breast practice was set top-down by the medical director. The reasons for not including them early on in the strategy formulation was to avoid early resistance to change and prevent the strategy being disseminated outside the organization before its adoption. There was more managerial control (top down) and less clinical control (bottom up) of the strategy concept and adoption stage, but with a clear clinician engagement plan at the diffusion stage. The latter included external and internal clinician championship, knowledge transfer (brokering) from inside and outside the organization (Sousa 2008; Cillo 2005).

The innovation diffusion stage is considered the stage when power dynamics are shifted from top down to bottom up. Senior leaders continue to lead on the strategic vision, but they should also share the leadership with clinical leaders; the latter could then play the role of middle-managers (clinic directors/leads/facilitators), subject matter experts and strategy implementers (Currie and Spyridonidis 2018). Organizational senior leaders were persistent in their leadership and supported the innovation movement to the diffusion stage, including offering project management, commercial, marketing and investment support (Waldman and Bass 1991). The latter was important so that the clinical leaders could focus on implementation of innovations, peer engagement and driving more business through.

The speed that innovations were expected to be delivered by the organization was considered to be overambitious by doctors and internal staff alike. Doctors needed more time for some innovation ideas to mature, they wanted to see a general buy-in consensus from peers, some wanted to pilot innovations followed by their adoption. This resulted in some innovations being delayed or not diffused at the time of the program end. Representative innovation examples included the patient reported outcome measures and the patient registries. Doctors struggled to agree on the type of patient reported outcome measure (PROM) to adopt and they also struggled to see the value gained from the registry adoption.

In both of those scenarios and in the case of clinical trials and patient portal, the time was very rushed to achieve full implementation and diffusion. The decision was made to move those innovations to version 2 of the innovation programme strategy in the year to follow.

The speed of innovation was so rapid at the diffusion and implementation stage that required strong managerial and senior medical leadership support (some top-down support). The latter helped guide doctors and internal staff during the implementation process. Good and stable leadership was demonstrated through staff engagement. Staff were kept motivated, inspired and on track to deliver the innovations in the required time frame. It also avoided scope creep which is a key risk in complex innovation processes. The bravery and agility of the senior leaders was shown in that certain innovation were moved to phase 2 of the program (year 2/version 2), in order to have more time to co-create with front-line clinicians across all global businesses.

The difficulty that doctors and internal staff faced was the lack of protected time to train in the delivery of the innovations. They also struggled with ambidexterity in terms of being able to deliver on the innovation strategy at the same time as dealing with business as usual. A solution to the complex and chaotic innovation process was the formation of workstreams which had operational and middle management support, tracing the actions and project managing the workstreams. There was agile and matrix working between workstreams to ensure there was enough capacity and support at all times. Leadership was shared with middle management who had the overall responsibility for their workstream. There was also a diverse collection of stakeholders in each workstream who brought unique skill sets and leadership capabilities so that they have a positive impact on innovation outcomes.

Clinical leadership was distributed and strengthened in the middle of the program year, with the formation of a breast clinical reference group (CRG), consisting of 6 clinicians including breast oncologists, breast cancer surgeons and a radiologist specialising in breast cancer. The CRG continued the education and knowledge reinforcement of peers around radiotherapy techniques, initiated radiotherapy plan reviews, and set up a weekly breast multidisciplinary meeting for any doctor who wanted to refer patients for discussion. The doctors who accepted to become members of the CRG were the ones whose values were totally aligned with those of the company. They were also strong advocates for the proposed innovations (Waldman and Bass 1991). The CRG members were selected for their unique agency skills and for their work as hybrid doctors, meaning doctors who could also lead and manage change at large scale, alongside their clinical responsibilities. There is evidence that hybrid doctors can bridge the gap between innovation and healthcare delivery and can drive innovation which is scalable and sustainable (Siribaddana et al. 2019). Medical doctors in leadership positions can enable better healthcare outcomes, engage clinical teams and improve organizational culture (Clay-Williams et al. 2017).

There were innovations which were not ready to be diffused at the 12th month mark such as genomics, registries, clinical trials, PROMs and the Cardio-Oncology service. However, the foundations were created and service aspects were adopted, with the prospect of developing further through more national and international collaborations. Given that those innovations were naturally complex, they required more networking and peer support before an implementation plan was drawn.

Some feedback received from the clinical reference group and other middle managers was the following:

> Certain innovations should have been labelled as phase 2 innovation from the beginning, with phase 1 being the immediate priorities or 'low hanging fruit'
> **Business development 1, Centre leader 2, CRG Director**

> As phase 1 innovations got diffused, they would naturally fall off the wheel and others would be added
> **Service improvement manager**

> By keeping all innovations on the wheel at the same time, was counterproductive for some, it didn't give enough opportunity for people to learn as they went along
> **Centre leader 1, Radiographer 1, Physicist**

There is a need to train and develop more doctor leaders who can cross their professional boundaries and lead within complex healthcare organizations. The positive impact of clinical leaders lies in knowledge brockering, maintaining resilience within teams and inspiring innovation across healthcare organizations and systems. What this innovation case demonstrated is that healthcare systems which are clinically well-led, are led 'bottom-up' with top-down support and are more able to align their business strategy with clinical need. Doctor involvement in senior leadership teams can ensure the delivery of high-quality care in a compassionate and holistic way.

Piloting the innovations in one or more areas followed by a plan to scale up the innovations was a tactical approach to protect the organization from risky innovations. Leaders ensured that they shared the learnings from the innovation process, celebrated the successes and created a culture of continuous innovation within the organisation. By the end of the 12-month period of intense innovation implementation, the innovation process was embedded in the day-to-day business across the organization (Millar et al. 2018). Innovation was no longer a siloed activity; instead, a framework for innovation implementation was constructed and supported by all stakeholders including the doctors. The implementation framework was also utilised in other markets where the company operated.

Innovation commercialisation and marketing became more pronounced at the 'scale up' (sustainability) stage of innovation, the time when innovations were spread to other oncological specialties (urology, hematology) and to other markets. This stage of innovation required a different leadership style, that is a more transactional (top-down) leadership style, in order to ensure the desired performance and benefit outcomes of the innovation strategy were achieved at scale and in a timely manner. This leadership style adopted by the senior leaders in the organization were balanced by the inspirational and transformational leadership style required in the earlier stages of innovation adoption and diffusion in those respective specialties and markets.

Clinician incentivisation featured strongly in the implementation phase of the innovation program. Clinician champions were incentivised to deliver on certain innovations through the form of financial reward (bonus) based on the number of patient referrals who would be treated with a specific technique or through a specific service. Clinician incentivisation also included ongoing training in radiotherapy techniques (continuous professional development) and the use of innovative resources to optimise their work efficiency and accuracy.

The senior leadership oversight was critical in this stage of intense implementation which helped to manage and roll with people's resistance to change; target individual doctors with education, training and exposure to key opinion leaders and champions; establish champions and innovation advocates; advertise and publish benefits through literature, interviews and adverts; present the innovations at conferences and events; representing key national and international meetings. The leadership team remained persistent to the innovation agenda. Their perseverance paid off and pushed more doctors to come on board and adopt the innovations.

The continuous oversight role of the senior leadership at the implementation phase of the innovation program was to ensure that innovations are constantly challenged and refined according to the needs of the patient population, the market and the organization. The clinical teams sometimes experienced some conflict between what the management leaders pushed as innovation agenda and what the patient population actually needed. The key opinion leaders and the breast CRG were the link between the company management and the patients (end receivers). Patient experience was evaluated through multiple formal and informal patient forums within the centres. This is a good example of how the organization top-down leadership tried to meet population needs through a bottom-up leadership approach. The top-down transactional approach earlier on in the adoption phase and later on in the sustainability phase of the innovation program was balanced by the more bottom-up transformational leadership in the diffusion and implementation phases of the innovation program and this balance helped push the successful implementation of most of the 24 innovations in 12 months.

4.5 Balancing Innovation, Transformation and Risk

The Healthcare market is competitive and healthcare organizations are forced to innovate often disruptively in order to gain competitive advantage. Within such a volatile and unpredictable environment, healthcare organizations need to balance the risk of innovation with being responsive enough to patient needs (Trastek et al. 2014). At the same time, clinical leaders should ensure that innovation is done with patient safety in mind and there is no conflict between innovation and business as usual.

A strong sense of purpose and alignment with the organization values was a unanimous feeling amongst people in this innovation program and 'innovation' was one of the organizational values. This is important as it meant that innovation is a 'business as usual' activity whose process is embedded in the workplace and every day. The organization's own model of care is about innovation for improving patient quality of care and patient outcomes.

The strong and agile team working amongst front-line teams, middle managers and centre leaders was key to the success of the innovation program. This was partly due to the fact that the teams within centres were small and all reported to one centre manager. However, the whole UK leadership team played a role in supporting middle managers and front-line leaders in the innovation process. Matrix working between the quality and human resource teams ensured governance and performance oversight respectively. Regular stand-up type of reporting and longer Kaizen type of events enabled people to brainstorm for innovation within their teams. There was clear accountability for innovation outcomes and people had an opportunity to reach out for resource support and mentorship.

Standardized quality and patient experience dashboards meant that people had access to the same data at all times, to be able to monitor innovation deliverables, refine and continuously improve services.

Centre leaders and the UK leadership team felt that disruptive innovation and patient safety are not mutually exclusive and that a well-led innovation approach can mitigate safety risks whilst innovating. Training on quality improvement methodologies and creating the space to share learnings from successful and failed innovation processes between centres was key for the majority of stakeholders interviewed.

The need for some workforce slack was identified by the centre leaders as key, to enable people to work on innovations without compromising their day role. This was probably one significant downside of this ambitious program of work. One area which could have been better planned early on in the program is the avoidance of running parallel projects with the same clinical and operational leaders. Although it was financially attractive to have same capable individual leaders owning multiple workstreams of work, this was unsustainable in the long-term and an area of reflection in preparation for the phase 2 of the program. Training more clinical and operational leaders to lead on individual workstreams of work was the strategy devised for the next phase of the program.

4.6 Why Did the Innovation Program Succeed

The overall perception of the innovation strategy adoption and diffusion by the various stakeholders, was that it partially succeeded. This is because not all innovations were diffused and implemented 12 months after the strategy creation. On the other hand, what the organization has definitely succeeded in creating, is an effective model of innovation diffusion success that could be replicated in other specialties and in other markets—something like a blueprint of innovation.

> The innovation strategy was a 100% success because it created a movement and brought clinicians much closer to the executive and middles management teams than ever before
> **Service improvement manager**

Drawing from stakeholder interviews and from observations made throughout the innovation process, we have summarised the lessons learned from this case and split them into: 'what's worked and why, for whom and under what circumstances' and 'what did not work and why, for whom and under what circumstances':

What works

- Management and clinicians working closer together using a balanced top-down and bottom-up approach at different stages in the innovation process. In particular, a top-down directional or transactional leadership style was appropriate at the ideation (concept of innovation) and adoption stages of innovation. This is due to innovation complexity which clinicians find difficult to navigate and which often conflicts with their standard way of practice. Market threats and opportunities are also commercial aspects which clinicians are not usually involved with and need direction. Senior leader top-down support can maximise the chance for innovation being commissioned. On the other hand, a more

bottom-up or transformational leadership approach is more appropriate in the later stages of innovation, when clinical champions of innovation drive innovation diffusion and implementation. An agile leadership style shifting between transactional and transformational leadership can optimize adoption, diffusion and implementation of innovations and can pave the way to scaling up innovation.
- Ownership of innovation within teams can boost sense of achievement and satisfaction and stakeholder engagement should be done early, allowing for co-creation of innovation.
- Organizational culture is essential in driving risk-taking behaviour and optimising peoples' courage and bravery to consider the adoption and diffusion of disruptive innovations. A relationship of trust between clinical leaders and the organization, builds on the clinical leader perception that they would be rewarded for their efforts. There are various incentivization models from financial (bonuses), to knowledge building (continuous professional development), to promotion and working practice improvements (digital tools, time and space for innovation, supportive services). Such perception is likely to motivate clinical leaders to adopt innovation and support their diffusion (Asgari et al. 2008).
- Data analytics should be embedded in the innovation process in order to capture the voice of the customer and the end—user experience.
- Clinical engagement needs a combination of visionary leadership (what can be achieved which will make care better for patients) and appropriate incentivization (what's in it for me).
- Greater clinical leader involvement and autonomy in day to day running of centres, would make clinicians appreciate the operational and governance aspects of the

business and also help them re-align their values with those of the organisation.
- Clinician perception of the innovation based on their knowledge and experience could determine whether clinical leaders will be 'early adopters' or 'laggards'. Targeting the early adopters and provided that there is strong leadership from their part, is a good tactical way of creating positive peer pressure hence achieving the required outcome from innovations.
- Innovation in healthcare needs to be clinically led and delivered and the aim should be the earlier engagement of key opinion leaders into the strategy formulation and communication.
- Clinical reference groups comprise a critical mass of clinical leaders in a specific subject that can be tasked with knowledge transfer, training and education of peers; advocating for innovation, driving the evaluation of innovation implementation and publishing the results.
- Integrated care should be maximised with the involvement of different clinical leaders including nurses, doctors, therapists and other professionals in a multidisciplinary team working style (distributed leadership).
- Platform—based innovations whereby a standardized innovation process can be applied to other healthcare areas and markets can enable innovation diffusion and sustainability. The economic benefit of scale is maximized and the risk is minimised by doing so.

What does not work

- Lack of clinician internal motivation to make changes in practice can be a significant blocker to innovation diffusion success. Alignment between clinical and

management leaders is key in terms of values and purpose of innovation, but clinician incentivisation still needs to be considered. Although this means financial rewards for some people, others would value the opportunity to receive training and credentialling in innovations and also engage with commercial partners for the purpose of clinical research.
- Scope creep and change in the innovation narrative are potential barriers to innovation diffusion and implementation, which can result in management and clinical leader disengagement. The diversity of innovations and the pressure to implement them all within a short period of time created pressure within the operational teams and resulted in some innovations not being implemented or their implementation being delayed.
- Innovation silos in healthcare without the power of internal and external partnerships or the integration of clinical specialties could have a negative impact in the diffusion of innovations. This was observed in the case of the more complex innovations such as genomics, where there was lack of standardised practice amongst clinicians.
- Innovation which is not linked to quality outcomes and the improvement of patient experience poses risks to the organization and the sustainability of innovation. A clear benefit realisation plan with specific and measurable clinical quality outcomes which go beyond the innovation financial benefits is likely to entice clinician leaders to support.
- Evaluation of innovation implementation should be embedded in the innovation process and be introduced early on the process. Healthcare innovation which is not outcome focused and is not evaluated in terms of its impact to end-users, staff and the organization may not sustain.

- Power differences between the medical director and the frontline leaders could have had a damaging effect in the diffusion of innovation. The use of positional power rather than motivational power by the senior leaders(s) to achieve innovation spread, can result in front-line leader disengagement. The role of the senior clinical leader is to act as the facilitator of innovation and change, learning from experimentation, sharing the learnings, distributing leadership and being the 'interpretation' agent between front-line and senior management when it comes to the change agenda (Edmonstone 2009). The medical director mitigated against that risk through the inclusion of international key opinion leaders and through leadership distribution to the clinical reference group.

References

Asgari A et al (2008) The relationship between transformational leadership behaviors, organizational justice, leader-member exchange, perceived organizational support, trust in management and organizational citizenship behaviors. Eur J Sci Res 23(2):227–242

Berkhout AJ, Hartmann D, van der Duin P, Ortt R (2006) Innovating the innovation process. Int J Technol Manag 34(3/4):390–404

Bessant J, Tidd J (2013) Managing innovation. www.innovationportal

Blizzard JL, Klotz LE (2012) A framework for sustainable whole systems design. Des Stud 33:456–479

Bolwijn P, Kumpe T (1990) Manufacturing in the 1990s productivity, flexibility and innovation. Long Range Plan 23(4):44–57. https://doi.org/10.1016/0024-6301(90)90151-S

Burgess N, Currie G (2013) The knowledge brockering role of the hybrid middle level manager: the case of healthcare. Br J Manag 24:S132–S142

Cillo P (2005) Fostering market knowledge use in innovation: the role of internal brokers. Eur Manag J 23(4):404–412

Clay-Williams R et al (2017) Medical leadership, a systematic narrative review: do hospitals and healthcare organisations perform better when led by doctors? BMJ Open 2017(7):e014474. https://doi.org/10.1136/bmjopen-2016-014474

Crevani L, Lindgren M, Packendorff J (2007) Shared leadership: a post-heroic perspective on leadership as a collective construction. Int J Leaders Stud 3(1):40–67

Crompton-Phillips A (2020) Spreading at scale: a practical leadership model for change. NEJM Catalyst 1(1)

Currie G, Spyridonidis D (2018) Sharing leadership for diffusion of innovations in professionalised settings. Hum Relat 1–25

de Ven V (2017) The innovation journey: you can't control it but you can learn to maneuvre it. Innov Organiz Manag 19(1):39–42

Dopson S, FitzGerald L, Ferlie E et al (2002) No magic targets! Changing clinical practice to become more evidence-based. Health Care Manag Rev 27(3):35–47

Edmonstone J (2009) Clinical leadership: the elephant in the room. Int J Health Plan Manag 24:290–305

Fukofuka S, Lokke DT (2015) OCTAPACE and organizational resilience: a correlational study. OJBMR 4(1):1–10

Glew J (2002) Whole systems thinking in health and social care. Woodville consultancy

Hao B, Feng Y, Iles P, Brown N (2017) Rethinking distributed leadership: dimensions, antecendents and team effectiveness. Leaders Organiz Dev J 38(2)

Jones B, Horton T, Walburton W (2019) The improvement journey. The Health Foundation

Livi L, Meattini I, Marrazzo L et al (2015) Accelerated partial breast irradiation using intensity-modulated radiotherapy versus whole breast irradiation: 5-year survival analysis of a phase 3 randomised controlled trial. EJC 51(4):451–463

Millar CJM, Groth O, Mahon JF (2018) Management innovation in a VUCA world: challenges and recommendations. California Manag Rev 61(1):5–14

Money AG, Barnett J, Kuljis J et al (2011) The role of the user within the medical device design and development process: medical device manufacturers' perspectives. BMC Med Inform Decis Mak 11:15

Papanicolas I, Mossialos E, Gundersen A et al (2019) Performance of UK National Health Service compared with other high income countries. BMJ 367:l6326

Shah SGS, Robinson I (2007) Benefits of and Barriers to involving users in medical device technology development and evaluation. Int J Technol Assess Healthc 23(1):131–137

Siribaddana P, Hewapathirana R, Sahay S, Jayatilleke A, Vajira HW (2019) 'Hybrid Doctors' can fast track the evolution of a sustainable e-health ecosystem in low resource contexts: the Sri Lankan experience. In: International medical informatics association (IMIA). IOS Press. https://doi.org/10.3233/SHTI190448

Sousa M (2008) Open innovation models and the role of knowledge brokers. www.ikmagazine.com

Trastek VF et al (2014) Leadership models in health cared: a case for servant leadership. Mayo Clin Proc 89(3):374–381

Van Der Duin P, Ortt R, Kok M (2007) The cyclic innovation model: a new challenge for a regional approach to innovation systems? Eur Plan Stud 15(2):195–215. https://doi.org/10.1080/09654310601078689

Waldman DA, Bass BM (1991) Transformational leadership at different phases of the innovation process. J High Technol Manag Res 2(2):169–180

West M et al (2017) Caring to change: how compassionate leadership can stimulate innovation in healthcare. The King's Fund

5

Using Learnings to Make a Model of Innovation Success

Abstract In order to design a model of leadership for innovation success, we drew from innovation practices from the two innovation case studies and in particular, what's worked well in terms of leadership, what could have been done differently, the barriers and enablers to innovation from a leadership perspective. We collected lessons learned through ethnography, participant observations and semi-structured interviews and common themes were extracted which informed the creation of a new preliminary model of healthcare innovation success.

5.1 The Preliminary Model of Innovation

The data collected from both innovation cases have been broken down into themes, summarizing barriers and enablers to innovation diffusion from a leadership perspective.

From the themes, we drew the commonalities from both case studies in terms of leadership enablers and barriers to innovation success.

The first commonality in both case studies, is the importance of a *shared vision and purpose within healthcare organizations* which is driven top down primarily, from the executive team to the front-line workforce. A shared vision is accompanied by organizational values which should resonate with all employees. Both organizations have 'innovation' high in their agendas; the NHS organization has 'innovation' in its mission statement and as part of its key objectives for delivering its vision to be a national and international leader in healthcare; the private organization features 'innovation' as one of its values. The difference between the two organizations is the fact that the private one had embedded 'innovation' into its culture and featured in its day-to-day business. On the contrary, the NHS organization had not invested on developing a more entrepreneurial culture, despite the fact that it truly believed that 'innovation' was the way forward. This key difference played a critical role in the innovation outcomes in both studies, as discussed further below.

Once a clear organizational vision and purpose is defined which features 'innovation', *a clear and plausible innovation strategy* needs to be co-designed with key stakeholders. In case 2, the medical director defined and designed the innovation strategy which was quickly endorsed by the organization with no resistance. The strategy was aligned with the overall purpose and mission of the organization and was shared with the front-line workforce and clinical leaders in a top-down approach. The strategy was plausible and had clear benefits which were well-defined and with a plan to measure at regular intervals. Innovation was promoted within the context of the organizational broader strategy and therefore became acceptable from the internal workforce very quickly. The doctors and referrers to the organization made up the external workforce and the majority if not all of the leadership efforts were spent to involve and empower clinical leaders into the innovation program. There was a whole organizational response to this effect.

The private organization could have done better in terms of scoping the innovation strategy with front-line staff, to ensure that the innovation strategy aligned with the operational capabilities needed during its implementation. The vision to implement 24 innovations in a space of one year was too ambitious and it conflicted with business-as usual activities. In addition, the lack of clinical leader involvement at the start of the innovation process may have resulted in the lack of diffusion or delayed diffusion for some of the innovations.

The innovation strategy was less clear in the NHS case study which hindered the implementation of the proposed innovation. There was also no defined digital strategic roadmap where the proposed innovation could have been part of. As a result, people within and outside the organization (industry and academic partners) found that the purpose of the proposed innovation did not align with the broader organizational purpose. This made it more difficult for external commissioners to buy-in to its usefulness and long-term sustainability. The learnings from the failed innovation in the NHS led to the re-definition of the Trust's innovation strategy, enhancing the chances of future innovation success.

Clinical championship was essential in both innovation cases. Both innovations were well championed by a medical leader, who managed to articulate a compelling vision for the future model of care. In the private sector case, the senior medical leader ensured that the strategy was plausible and that it met a clinical unmet need as well as a gap in the market. In addition, the medical leader secured executive support and resources before proceeding to the implementation of the strategy. In the NHS case, the medical leader articulated a compelling case for change which was theoretically supported by the executives but there was no secure execution plan and resources for the strategy implementation. The lack of a broader stakeholder involvement, including more clinical leaders, made the case for change even more difficult to execute. This resulted in the innovation being perceived as an extra workload, on top of business-as-usual activity, lacking facilitation from senior management in terms of offering discretionary time and space for clinicians to innovate and lacking organizational commitment to sustain the innovation.

Clinician incentivization was an enabler in getting clinical leaders closer to the innovation program in the case 2 and eventually making them key members of the innovation strategy moving forward. It required a degree of investment from the executive leadership team in terms of offering technological tools and dedicated workforce to support clinician workload. It also meant that clinicians were rewarded through a bonus-based scheme for the innovation work they did, as innovations brought more patient referrals into their clinical practice. The lack of an incentivization plan for clinicians in case 1 was a barrier to getting them invest time and energy in supporting the innovation. Clinician incentivization in this specific case would have taken the form of dedicated time in clinicians' job plan to work on the innovations and dedicated organizational resources to implement and scale their innovations. If the latter was provided, clinicians would have been more likely to support the adoption of the innovation for the purpose of improving patient care. The lack of clinician incentivization in the latter case contributed heavily to the lack of innovation endorsement and adoption.

Business case plausibility in terms of the presence of quantitative data for evidence of the innovation benefits was an important enabler for achieving stakeholder buy-in in both cases. In case 2, a plausible business case meant that there was a forecasted and clear financial benefit as early as one year after strategy implementation, which made it easier for the company to invest into the strategy straight away. The *culture of experimentation* that characterized the private organization meant that they were more likely to bear the investment risk in the prospect of a higher prospective financial gain. Organizational leaders promoted learning through experimentation and failure, which made it easier for staff to become engaged in innovation activities. The culture of psychological safety and the acceptance of failure by senior management, meant that people consistently brought forward new ideas for implementation and there was already a track record of innovation diffusion within the organization. The NHS business case also had a clear long-term benefit evaluation plan, which demonstrated a healthy return on investment. However, the organization was reluctant to bear the risk and invest on the innovation. The absence of a culture of experimentation and risk-taking behaviour in the organization, led to the lack of investment for the proposed innovation despite its long-term and sustainable benefits.

The private organization *engaged key opinion leaders early on in the innovation* process and using a repeated knowledge transfer and reinforcement strategy to make the case for change and remove resistance to change from clinical leaders. In the NHS case, the digital innovation had a plausible business case but there were no key opinion leaders engaged to share their knowledge and experience on the proposed innovation. The lack of key opinion leaders, peer and non-peer support, in combination with the lack of Trust resources to support innovation implementation and commercialization, meant that the innovation did not receive commissioner support and failed to be adopted.

End user acceptance was perceived as an enabler in the digital innovation case in the NHS and was rated highly by commissioners. However, end user acceptance alone and without top-down support did not drive success. On the other hand, end user acceptance was variable in the case of the private sector innovation model but there was strong top-down support. This example demonstrates the importance of top-down leadership in changing clinician and patient behaviour but only when end users are willing to lead and champion change at the same time.

Patient and public involvement (PPI) was well embedded from the early stages of innovation in case 1, unlike case 2. PPI was highly rated by NHS commissioners and was greatly appreciated by patients and the innovation team alike in case 1, as it brought very useful insights into the project implementation plan. In the private sector case, PPI did not take place during the creation of the innovation strategy or during its implementation, but this was not detrimental to the innovation outcomes. The technical nature of many of the innovations made them hard to explain to patients and get their understanding. Other innovations were 'nice to have' additions to the existing services which none of the patients would object to. A good example of those were the exercise and wellbeing facilities in the centres. Innovations to improve the technical aspects of treatment delivery were again not appropriate to share or negotiate with patients. The set-up of a patient experience forum with the task of measuring and reporting patient experience outcomes following the diffusion of innovations, compensated for the upfront lack of patient and public involvement in case 2.

Partnerships were very important in the NHS innovation process, consisting of academic and industry partners.

It was important for the NHS organization to have trusted partners early on in the process, because it meant that the risk was shared amongst partners and made the case for change more likely to be sustained if all partners were ready to commit to transforming care. Within the partnership, the NHS Trust would offer useful data around the 'before and after' state of care, which partners would use for the technical execution and the evaluation aspects of the model. The partners offered commercial and academic expertise which strengthened the case for change and inspired confidence in terms of the innovation's scale up capability. Partnership working was well received by the commissioners of the national innovation funding competition. However, there were concerns around the business and technical capabilities of the NHS organization under study, which would have been necessary in order to execute the innovation. In the private healthcare case study, partnerships were formed between organizational executives, clinical leaders and international key opinion leaders for the purpose of delivering the innovation program. In addition, the company sought a number of industrial partnerships in order to deliver the digital aspects of the innovation program. The company operated with 'partnership' as one of its core values, so the involvement of several vendors in the execution of the strategy was part of day-to-day activities. Partnerships had already been built into the internal innovation capability of the organization rather than being done as an exception, which was more so the case with the NHS case study. The strong partnering culture of the organization was catalytical as much in the early stage of innovation adoption as in the later stages of innovation implementation and sustainability.

Clinical leaders as enablers of innovation are best placed to facilitate communication channels between executive boards and front-line clinicians within organizations

(Bourgeois and Brodwin 1984). Our experience in case 2 (private healthcare) is that the senior medical leader in the organization initially took the role of the executive top-down strategist, spearheading the innovation program and gaining organizational support. This transactional leadership style led to the innovation model being launched and implementation starting at pace and across all centres simultaneously. Subsequently, the senior medical leader took the role of the meso-level manager and facilitator of communication between front-line staff, clinical leaders and the executive team during the intense implementation phase. At that stage, the senior medical leader used a more transformation leadership style in order to inspire change. The driving of key opinion leader and clinician engagement happened at the same time as the strategy was implemented rather than sequentially. Roadshows, conference events and literature development by the senior medical leader strengthened the argument for change. These activities were used as a means of showcasing the strategy and its outcomes in order to motivate clinicians to adopt the innovations across all the centres. Distributed leadership to the clinical reference group was key in the diffusion, implementation but also sustainability and growth of the innovation program. What was also observed at the later stages in the innovation process is that the senior medical leader reverted back to the initial transactional style of leadership in the effort to achieve clinical standardisation across the board and address any residual resistance to change. We also found that the role of the non-clinical middle managers in the centres became critical at the later stages of innovation. They supported the continuous clinician engagement and offered support to their front-line teams so that they could sustain innovation. Expanding the network of clinicians and collaborating with international leaders within and outside the group at the diffusion and implementation stages ensured continuous support to drive the innovation forward to other markets.

In case 1 (NHS), the medical leader played the role of the front-line clinical innovator. The clinical innovator spearheaded the innovation, led an innovation team, the partnership model for innovation and the patient-public involvement. However, the innovator lacked the hierarchical power within the organization to make innovation happen. Unlike case 2, where the senior medical leader was also a member of the executive team, in case 1, the medical leader was a clinician with no senior management duties. As a result, the leadership style of the innovator was mostly transformational, in order to enable clinician motivation and engagement rather than transactional and directional. It is important to note, that the lack of top-down support in case 1 in terms of internal resource allocation, clinician incentivization and commercial capabilities, made it difficult for the medical leader to convince clinicians to enact change. Similarly, the lack of top-down support was perceived by the commissioners as one of the biggest risks for the spread of the proposed innovation. Without spread, the innovation would not have delivered on the return of investment as suggested in the business case.

Power relationships played an important role in the final outcome of both innovation case studies. The private case study demonstrated the need for the senior medical leader to have an agile leadership style using a top-down transactional approach in the early phase of innovation (top-down senior medical sponsor during ideation and adoption), a more transformational and engaging style during the middle stages of implementation (post-adoption), reverting back to the transactional style in the late phase of implementation and sustainability. The innovator's meso-level leader and facilitator role during the early stages of implementation bridged the gap between front-line clinicians and executive management, in terms of clinical communication, shared understanding, shared learning and alignment to same goals. A collaboration between front-line clinicians and organizational management is very important to ensure that there is alignment between these two culturally diverse groups (Doherty 2013). The senior medical leader was the enabling agent between the entrepreneurial executive team and the operational front-line, which pushed innovations from ideas to execution, at pace. This occurred primarily through the senior medical leader's strategy of engaging key opinion leaders, the development of clinical networks (clinical reference group) and matrix working involving centre staff, clinicians, international experts, innovation partners and the executive team (Arena and Uhl-Bien 2016; Uhl-Bien and Marion 2009).

In case 1, the medical leader had no executive positional power but had power over the other clinical colleagues (the non-innovators). The fact that the innovator designed the innovation idea without any co-creation from peers, shifted the ownership of the innovation to the innovator alone. Any effort from the innovator to engage other medics failed to result in any supportive engagement from them. Unlike medics, the nurses and radiographers in the department were supportive of the innovation and willing to pilot the new model of care.

The proposed leadership in innovation model in Fig. 5.1 is a preliminary model that represented the leadership enablers and barriers from the two case studies.

This cyclical innovation model represents the dynamic and complex process of innovation within complex healthcare organizations. It represents innovation as a continuous process which the organizations need to invest on in terms of senior leadership, operational management and supportive resources.

5 Using Learnings to Make a Model of Innovation ...

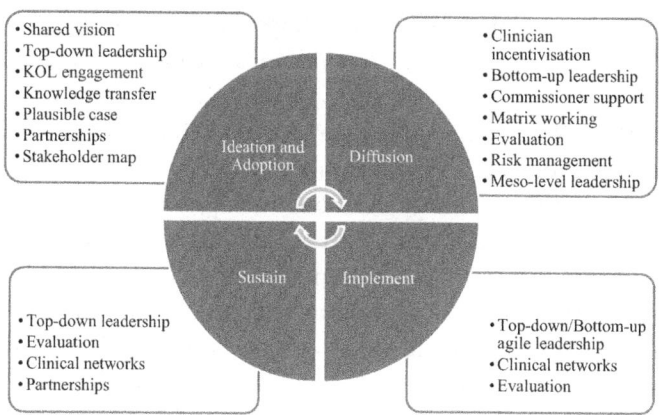

Fig. 5.1 Leadership in innovation preliminary model for success

Healthcare organizations exist within a complex and volatile context of financial, technical and market instability. What this means for organizations is that they need to constantly evaluate their innovation strategy, drop innovations if they don't deliver value and introduce new ones. The ambiguous and unstable political, social and economical environment of the last three years has taught healthcare organizations that there is an urgent need to innovate and transform in order to disrupt and gain competitive advantage.

The building of new organizational capabilities requires strong strategic leadership top-down, an entrepreneurial organizational culture of risk-taking and a suitable organizational leadership structure. Senior medical leaders working with operational management and front-line leaders in a matrix style of working can lead to an agile way of working. There is also an emerging need to predict the future of healthcare, forecast clinical unmet need and demand of customers through data analytics and be one step ahead in terms of strategy and leadership to be able to survive at unpredictable times (Millar et al. 2018).

We believe that innovation adoption and diffusion cannot materialize without partnerships including clinician networks, patients, academia, commercial and other charitable partners. The type of partnership will depend on the organization type, whether public or private and whether the innovation strategy is about new products, new services or both. Academic partners are key actors whatever the organization or innovation strategy due to their skillful resources in evaluating innovations. Patient and public involvement should be an integral component in any healthcare innovation process. Measuring patient experience and other innovation outcomes is key to ensuring that innovations add value to patients and the wider population, innovation benefits are shared, and innovation benefits are maximized and sustained.

References

Arena MJ, Uhl-Bien M (2016) Complexity leadership theory: shifting from human capital to social capital. People Strategy 39(2)

Bourgeois LJ, Brodwin DR (1984) Strategic implementation: five approaches to an elusive phenomenon. Strateg Manag J 5:241–264

Doherty J (2013). Strengthening clinical leadership in hospitals. In: Municipal Services Project Policy Brief

Millar CJM, Groth O, Mahon JF (2018) Management innovation in a VUCA world: challenges and recommendations. California Manag Rev 61(1):5–14

Uhl-Bien M, Marion R (2009) Complexity leadership in bureaucratic forms of organizing: a meso model. Management Department Faculty Publications, 38

6

Model Validation in Real-Time —*A Case Study*

Abstract Leadership plays an important role in enabling innovation adoption and diffusion within healthcare organizations. In healthcare settings, innovation diffusion depends on individual leadership behaviours and organisational culture, as demonstrated in (Brown et al. 2014). Innovation leaders have a great role to play in empowering teams to share ideas and knowledge, through ensuring trust and collaboration, work autonomy and through incentivization methods such as salary recognition, training and/or internal promotion opportunities (Kremer et al. 2019). Innovation behaviour within organizations depends as much on individual characteristics such as internal motivation, as on group support, top management support and the organizational culture of creativity and entrepreneurship (Kuratko et al. 2014). Strong managerial and clinical leadership which is aligned with the broad vision of the organization (front line to board) constitutes a powerful enabler for innovation (Schoenfeldt and Jansen 1997). Our new model of innovation diffusion considers the leadership characteristics and activities that help innovation move from the ideation and adoption phase to the diffusion and implementation phase within complex healthcare organizations and through the lens of two real innovation case studies. We found that top-down transactional leadership is probably dominant in the ideation and adoption stage, when the innovation strategy is created and innovations need to get adopted. On the other hand, bottom-up clinical leadership and greater matrix working amongst stakeholders is required in the diffusion and implementation stage, leading the way to the implementation and scale up of innovations. An agile leadership approach with a combination of top-down power and bottom-up agency, including the expansion of clinical networks, prevail in the stages of innovation implementation and sustainability.

6.1 Application of the New Model in a New Context

To test and refine the model of leadership in innovation, we have applied this to a new case study of innovation within the context of an NHS Trust strategic transformation. The NHS Trust is the same organization where the digital innovation process took place in case 1, but the external environment has changed, leading to internal changes as well.

In terms of the new context, following the pandemic years, the NHS Reform strategy (NHS Confederation 2021) was published which advocates for more joined up care between secondary care providers, primary, community and social care as well as voluntary services. Partnerships amongst care providers is the key to the delivery of a more patient-centred care, aimed at improving population outcomes whilst reducing health inequalities. The establishment of Integrated Care Systems in April 2021 is challenging the financial and political status of NHS organizations. Integrated Care Systems are advocating and supporting investment in innovation adoption, diffusion and sustainability. Recent national innovation schemes which have being implemented include the NHS innovation accelerator, digital aspirants, integrated care records and global digital exemplars amongst others. Digital innovations alongside digital literacy and inclusion are also priorities of the government which collectively can help dampen the demand for acute hospital care and ensure that the NHS aligns well with the more developed and invested-on private healthcare systems.

Leadership during the pandemic has allowed for critical decision making around infection prevention and control, vaccination, digital communications, telecare, test and trace and has given rise to several digital and other innovations in healthcare. Some of those include remote monitoring solutions, virtual wards, lifestyle applications and rapid technology deployments including shared medical records. At the specific NHS Trust level, clinicians stepped up to support the peaks of the pandemic with modifications in their clinical protocols to ensure patient safety and equity of care. The pandemic has spearheaded a culture of innovation and an acceleration of the innovation process from idea to implementation happening at pace. The post-pandemic phase has found most NHS organizations financially depleted, with a tired workforce and a surge of physical and mental illness across working staff and patients. The uncertainty around the financial sustainability of NHS providers alongside the need to return to pre-pandemic state of services, has sparked innovation across healthcare systems.

The NHS Trust under study has refocused its strategy post-pandemic to work as part of an integrated care system with primary care, commissioners, acute organizations, community and social care. The new strategic leadership and governance structure consist of multiple workstreams covering urgent and emergency care, tertiary care and networks, people and culture, finance and estates, supportive services and digital transformation. Each workstream has a senior responsible officer (SRO) who is accountable to the system and who manages the workstream clinical leaders using a distributed leadership approach. The SROs are all members of the Trust's Chief Officer Group. The purpose of the workstreams is for them to lead the new integrated model of care and restore service function post-pandemic. Innovation in this context is encouraged to improve service access, quality, efficiency, effectiveness and equity in healthcare.

The workstream clinical leaders were elected from the existing seven group clinical directors (GCDs) of the Trust. The GCDs are members of the group triumvirates, which also include a group director of operations and a group director of nursing. The link between front line staff and the Chief Officers was through the triumvirate groups who managed the communication messages between the two parties.

The innovator in this case was the group clinical director for surgery who also led the innovations in the previous two cases. The innovator found similarities in the breast cancer service vision with that of private sector case (case 2) hence this was a good opportunity to apply the proposed leadership in innovation model. The only difference was in the context, with case 3 being a complex NHS organization with significant system influence and which competed for resources with other providers.

The Breast cancer service had consistently overperformed over the years due to strong clinical leadership on the frontline, but the pandemic had caused strain in the service. There was an opportunity to restore and transform the breast cancer service into one of the most profitable, innovative and sustainable services in the Trust. On the back of that vision, the NHS Long Term Plan advocated for early diagnosis of breast cancer, improvement in cancer care outcomes and the use of genomics and genetics to deliver personalized healthcare. The use of advanced diagnostic technologies (including Artificial Intelligence) to improve the speed and accuracy of breast mammograms and the development of community diagnostic hubs to increase patient access to diagnostic tests closer to patient communities, were on the top of the innovation agenda. Advancement of radiotherapy techniques and personalized surveillance were also key priorities, alongside the use of digital technology to boost patient self-management and virtual consultations. Breast cancer innovations in the private healthcare sector (case 2) spanned the whole breast cancer pathway, from diagnosis through to treatment and survivorship and were implemented in their majority; the NHS now followed with the same innovation themes and strategic direction.

> Breast cancer two-week wait and 31-day breast cancer standards were met during the pandemic due to the hard work of the teams on the ground, who flexed their working time and space to be able to deliver
> **Clinical Lead Breast Surgery**

> We had to adapt to a new working environment in the private sector facilities, our equipment was not in the same place and there was a whole new IT infrastructure built for us that we had to learn as well
> **Breast care nurse**

> It would be good to have a permanent home as a breast team that also includes radiology and pathology, at the moment we all work at different places and never see each other or talk to each other
>
> **Breast radiologist**

> We need more investment to create a world-class breast cancer service that people can access easily, without having to travel to several places to receive care
>
> **Consultant Breast surgeon**

> Access to genomic testing for all breast cancer patients who benefit is a 'must', there is huge variation in the genetic offerings across the country and is not fair for our patients
>
> **Consultant Clinical Oncologist**

The group clinical director had the vision of expanding and developing the end-to-end breast cancer pathways from patient diagnosis through to survivorship, using a whole system approach to change, similar to case 2. The trigger for the movement was the change in the political environment, with the development of the integrated care system (ICS) and the dependence on the system for funding. There was considerable scope for innovation which would earn the Trust competitive advantage as the bigger NHS Trust in the system and also as a tertiary cancer provider for the ICS. Becoming a lead Trust provider of regional breast cancer services would potentially attract more commissioner investment for research, innovation and technological development. Those triggers for innovation and change were similar to case 2 but the environment was different:

– the NHS Trust is a public body and employs its doctors and clinical leaders, unlike the private organization;

- the NHS Trust was financed with block payments at the time of the study, whereas the private organization was financed through private equity;
- there was more secured funding in the private organization as long as innovation business cases delivered on the investment.

The proposed series of innovations were similar to case 2 and included the following:

- Faster diagnosis hub facility in the community;
- Personalized Oncology pathways incorporating genetics and genomics for decision-making about treatment;
- An expansion of radiotherapy treatment offerings;
- Flexible surgical workforce to increase capacity;
- Expansion of the breast surgical workforce;
- The development of a complex Cancer MDT;
- A health and wellbeing offering for patients;
- A systematic collection of patient reported outcomes;
- A collection of supportive services including cardio-Oncology, lymphoedema, bone health, psychological support;
- A surgical training program;
- Dedicated e-referral pathways for suspected cancer.

The Senior Responsible Officer for the tertiary workstream was the Chief Strategy Officer for the Trust and accountable for the delivery of the Trust's strategic direction including breast cancer services. The challenge to the status quo and the delivery of the strategic direction in breast cancer services was set top down, by the chief strategist and SRO in the organization, due to the pressing need to align with the NHS Long Term Plan and expand this profitable and reputable service. The integrated care system also had a primary role to play in terms of defining the overall direction of the system and the SRO played a leading role in the ICS.

> We need to work together as a system and utilize all our resource capacity smartly and efficiently
>
> **Chief Strategy Officer**

The enabler of innovation was the group clinical director for surgery who played the role of the enabling link between the entrepreneurial and the operational aspect of the service. The clinical director in this case was the middle manager and facilitator of innovation who could translate the top-down strategic direction to a bottom-up clinical service proposition which resonated with front-line teams, led by the breast surgery clinical lead.

The innovator's role was distinct to the middle manager role (operational delivery) but both collaborated closely in order to implement the strategy. The experience of the group clinical director was key, having sponsored one large transformation project (case 2), flexing between executive leadership and middle management and enacting distributed leadership when necessary. Tactics that were successful in case 2, were adapted in this case, which included local peer to peer key opinion leader engagement, timely front-line participation and commissioner collaboration.

In this volatile and ambiguous environment, the role of the commissioners as drivers of the overall vision for innovation within integrated care systems was critical. The commissioning role of shaping the culture of innovation and organizational behaviours was evident in this case, as it eliminated the resistance to change and influenced competition between providers (Corrigan et al. 2013). It also drove collaborations between providers such as in the case of the community diagnostic hubs (primary − secondary − social care integration) and the health and wellbeing hubs (third sector). We saw in case 1 that the lack of commissioner support worked negatively when competing for the innovation fund. In case 2, the commissioning was controlled internally by the organization and was therefore not an issue. In case 3, commissioner involvement drove the vision and direction of innovation which in turn shaped the culture of experimentation in the organization.

> Community diagnostic hubs is the future of care and will enable the NHS Long Term Plan's ambition to diagnose 75% of all cancers at an early stage
> **Clinical Diagnostics Group Director**

The strong direction from the commissioner group, the ICS and the Trust led to the key opinion leaders and front-line staff (surgeons, oncologists, radiologists, nurses) very quickly becoming the followers of the innovation strategy, without a huge engagement effort. This is a good example of a top-down strategy, supported by resources and facilitated by meso-level leadership. The group clinical director (innovator) together with the breast surgery clinical lead and the chief strategy officer agreed on the proposed innovation agenda which was then unfolded at different levels:

- *System level with the development of Community Diagnostic Hub facility to include breast cancer diagnostics.* The strategic vision of the Trust has been completely aligned with that of the integrated care system and commissioners of cancer care: from 2028, an extra 55,000 people each year will survive for five years or more following their cancer diagnosis and three in four cancers (75%) will be diagnosed at an early stage (stage 1 and 2). Faster cancer diagnosis standards will be implemented to ensure that patients are told their diagnosis accurately and within maximum 28 days from referral, speeding up the time from what's currently 31 days. The timeline for completion of this project is longer-term, nevertheless the financial commitment and planning of the project started at the end of our study period. Matrix working between commissioners and service providers (multi-specialties) including a local university (for research purposes) and commercial partners, increased the complexity of the project and justified its lengthy timeline for completion.

- *Patient-level with personalized Oncology pathways incorporating genetics and genomics.* In the NHS, there was no commissioning for personalized genomic services and a recent business case presented was not supported by the cancer board. This demonstrates that lack of available funding and commissioning support is a major factor in the diffusion of innovation. However, there is work that has started by the genomic medicine service alliance (GMSA) in the region, with the vision of using genomics to guide therapeutic modalities in oncology. In the case of breast cancer, specialist commissioning is looking at risk stratifying patients according to their genetic and genomic profile so that a personalized diagnostic, therapeutic and surveillance approach is implemented. NHS England in collaboration with Health Education England and the GMSA are on track to implement a digital risk stratification tool for use in primary and secondary care.

- *Organizational level with Breast Surgery to increase capacity.* The lack of surgical capacity both in theatre space and personnel, led to a collaborative approach between the public and private sector during the covid-19 pandemic. This collaboration resulted in the vast majority of breast cancer patients having no delays in their diagnosis and surgical treatment, as they could have their diagnostic scans and operations in private facilities, using flexible NHS and private resources. Following a successful business case outcome, an extra two breast surgeons were employed by the Trust with plans to work flexibly with other surgeons within the system, utilizing all available theatre capacity across providers. Although the flexible workforce model was not met with support across the system, the Trust invested in the development of new theatre capacity through the building of modular theatres. A combined top-down and bottom-up leadership approach prevailed here with the front-line staff identifying the problem (capacity shortage), the meso-level clinical director responding with a workforce business case and proposed new strategy and the executive team investing in further resources to meet the needs of the specialty. The expansion of the breast surgical workforce saw more senior level clinicians in post to help with the increasing demand of the service, deal with the backlog of operations due to the pandemic and create an agile and resilient workforce across the system.

- *The development of a complex cancer multidisciplinary team meeting* was proposed and the proposal was met with general support. However, the idea implementation was a system-wide one and linked with the development of the Trust's electronic health record (EHR). The innovation timeline was delayed to coincide with the EHR development.

- *A health and wellbeing offering for patients* at any stage of their illness was led through the Macmillan Cancer Information team leading to the Living Well Beyond Cancer program. The program was commissioned through the system and in association with local cancer charities. Members of the breast cancer multidisciplinary group were invited to participate in the task and finish group in order to create a patient-initiated follow up program after patients completed treatment. This is an excellent example of a top-down, commissioner-supported program with distributed leadership for its implementation.

- *A systematic collection of patient-reported outcome measures* through the upcoming patient portal became another long-term project to be included in the Electronic Health Record implementation program.
- *A collection of supportive services* including cardio-Oncology, lymphoedema, bone health, psychological support, menopause was led through the engagement of various clinical leaders within and outside the organization (system partners). Matrix working and clinical networking helped to incorporate the right clinical champions with specialist interest in these specific clinical specialties. For example, a cardiologist with specialist interest in Cardio-Oncology led educational sessions for oncology professionals in the Trust and opened the referral pathway to this clinic. Equally, the recruitment of psycho-Oncologists and counsellors led to a comprehensive wellbeing offering for patients.
- *An innovative surgical skills training program* was set up in the post-pandemic phase, led by a consultant breast surgeon and key opinion leader, in collaboration with other surgical clinical leaders. The collaborative nature of this program, championed by clinicians with a special interest in medical education is the reason for this program success in its first round. In addition, all surgical clinical leaders had connections with the local universities and academic health science networks and others worked with commissioners or NHS England. The surgeon and key opinion leader helped raise the profile of the program and secured funding and other resources to continue running the program in a sustainable way. Moreover, clinical leaders and the NHS Trust had strong connections with commercial partners that supplied the technological resources such as imaging, software and robotic technology who also had a vested interest in the education program. The strong academic

and health science networking opened the doors for research opportunities with the Trust. Finally, clinical leaders ensured that the program was evaluated well in terms of user satisfaction and clinical effectiveness and the results were published. The ongoing evaluation activity of the program led to its continual review and refinement, ensuring its sustainability long-term.

- *A dedicated e-referral pathway* was created so that GPs could refer suspected breast cancer patients to the hospital surgical team quickly and effectively. A presentation made by the group clinical director and the surgical clinical lead to the GPs regarding breast cancer pathways during the pandemic, revealed that the existing referral needed to be reviewed to ensure it covered all eventualities and patient presentations. The post-pandemic period which revealed a large backlog of undiagnosed cancer patients made the timely provision of an accurate breast e-referral more of a priority for the system.

6.2 Lessons Learned from a Complex Leadership and Innovation Context

Lesson 1—The commissioners of innovation and system leadership

The unstable and competitive political and economical context played a very important role in the innovation outcomes of case 3. The NHS Reform dictated the way of working in terms of outward thinking as a system and moving away from inward thinking (Trust-led). All services needed to demonstrate value for the population rather for a specific cohort of patients served by the Trust and there was an emergent need to allocate resources efficiently and based on adding societal value for better population health. One of the reasons for the need for allocation efficiencies and reduction in waste was the uncertainty in terms of commissioning of services and moving away from payment-by-results into block payments. This change would have normally made the appetite to invest in innovation less. However, there was recognition that innovation would bring more technical and technological capability, would incentivize the workforce to work smarter, leveraging available and emerging technologies and would result in more efficient allocation of resources. NHS Trusts working within an integrated care system had to compete for innovation resources based on the value associated with those innovation. This made the evaluation of innovation implementation in terms of benefit realization even more critical.

Integrated care systems should learn from the pandemic which demonstrated the role of devolved leadership structures to the front-line leaders and meso level managers. Command and control was prominent top-down in terms of decisions to enact lockdowns and the stopping of elective surgical activity across the country whilst acute hospitals tackled covid. However, it was the combined effort of the front-line clinical leaders and middle management who enacted their business continuity protocols but also developed innovative care pathways, resulting in patients getting the right care at the right time.

Similarly, the role of system and network partnerships opened up new opportunities for collaboration to ensure timely patient care provision. A good example is the public NHS provider contract with the private sector for the provision of life-saving cancer surgery during the pandemic. Such collaboration which resulted in the fast diagnosis and treatment of NHS cancer patients in the private sector as well as the close-working of the NHS workforce with that of the private sector for serving the common purpose, was revolutionary and demonstrated the power of public—private partnerships.

Research and innovation acceleration became a prominent feature in the pandemic and post-pandemic era. Breast cancer and other cancer pathways became individualized, in order to ensure that the right patients were prioritised for the right treatments. In addition, innovations were introduced in the way surgical procedures were performed, using innovative technology, which speeded up the time from diagnosis to surgery. Finally, the approval of new radiotherapy and chemotherapy protocols was accelerated, which would have otherwise taken months or years to be adopted. Such clinical trial evidence was published and disseminated within days or weeks and the clinical community adopted the new practices very quickly. The wide adoption, diffusion and scale up of those innovative techniques based on the need at the time of the pandemic, has demonstrated their positive outcomes very quickly. Evaluation outcomes were done at scale and gave the confidence to clinicians to continue using those innovative techniques in the post pandemic period.

Lesson 2—Key opinion leader engagement
Another useful lesson learned from this case is that if key opinion leaders (KOLs) who are the legitimate and respected clinical representatives, worked together with top managers and commissioners to embed the clinical evidence for innovation to current processes, front-line leaders would be more likely to champion innovations leading to innovation diffusion and implementation.

What was also critical was the close relationship between meso-level management, operational managers and the KOLs, which is also highlighted in Powell and Davies (2016). The building of a trustworthy relationship between the group clinical director and operational management helped the implementation of innovations which were clinically led. The relationship between executive sponsors, commissioners and front-line clinical leaders was enhanced through the presence of a meso-level enabling team, led by the group clinical director.

The group clinical director was in the unique position of being closer to the front-line clinicians as member of the multi-disciplinary breast cancer team and also being part of the triumvirate group (meso-structure), reporting straight to the executive team. She was also involved at strategic level and was able to communicate in a 'bottom up' manner the needs of patients and clinicians. At the same time, she communicated top-down the strategic direction as set by the Trust.

Very important elements in the success of the innovation strategy were the following:

– The system had the power to set the direction for innovation change and the Trust had no alternative other than responding to this call.
– The Senior Responsible Officer and other Chief Officers were supportive of the strategic direction and the innovation plans.
– Funding was available as a system and commissioners were supportive, but there was still the need to prioritize innovations.
– An engaged front-line team which was well-led was an essential ingredient to make the innovation program a success.

Lesson 3—The role of the meso-level leader makes a difference

The clinical director of the surgical group was the champion of the innovation strategy and worked across the whole patient pathway (surgery and oncology). The breast cancer service innovation program was aligned with the integrated care system (ICS) strategy, was SRO led and the leadership of its implementation was distributed. The role of the group clinical director was best placed at the meso-level where it played the collaborative link between front line leaders and the SRO.

Early doctor engagement and enablement of the front-line subject matter experts took the strategy forward because it meant that there was a critical mass of clinician leaders who were empowered to push the innovation agenda forward. What's also important is that the group management team came closer to the front-line clinicians through the meso-level director to facilitate entrepreneurial ideas becoming operationalized. The meso-level director also drove the top-down engagement between the executive team and the front-line workforce, which had a positive impact on other surgical service innovation strategies within the same organization.

Lesson 4—Prioritizing innovations based on societal value

Going back to the breast service innovations, they represented a complete end to end pathway for breast cancer, from diagnosis through to survivorship. Unlike the case 2 strategy whereby the goal was to adopt and diffuse 24 innovations in 12 months, the focus on case 3 was limited to the services that would add most societal value in years 1 and 2.

Those innovations were around aspects of care that were either compromised during the pandemic (cancer diagnostics) or their implementation was delayed because of the pandemic (personalized care).

The narrow focus of the innovation strategy and the top-down drive of innovations meant that the project at year 1 was more achievable. In addition, the conflict between business as usual and innovation that we experienced with case 2, was not evident. Front-line clinical leaders with the support of the group clinical director and group manager, sponsored by the chief officers, broke down the innovations into time-limited chunks that were easily achievable. The involvement of front-line leaders and middle management in innovation was also factored in their job plans. This motivated clinical leaders further as they had the space and autonomy to think innovatively, they worked with teams to implement innovation and they saw quick results being delivered.

For example, within a couple of months of the innovation strategy being co-created and presented to the executive team, the business case for breast cancer surgical consultant expansion was approved and recruitment began. This boosted the morale of the front-line staff and increased their trust to the process. The Trust's Chief officers, the meso—level group, its front-line clinical leaders and the system worked in collaboration. In addition, there was visible innovation accountability at the Trust executive level as well as ownership of innovation at the clinical level.

The relationship building between front-line and executive teams increased the confidence on both sides to enter regular and direct conversations. This was an opportunity for executives to give the system direction and vision and the clinical leaders to respond from a clinical evidence base. This gave the opportunity for the executives to understand the challenges on the front line, link with other groups such as diagnostics and oncology to understand the interdependencies and refine the strategic view of the breast service. The front-line clinical leaders also felt that their challenges were heard at the top level of the organization.

The Trust executives were accurately advised by the clinical leaders regarding the proposed innovative solutions and on how to improve and grow Trust services, in collaboration with system partners. The clinical leaders were encouraged by the executive team to connect with their counterparts from neighbouring Trusts and engage in conversations about creating a single regional breast service. This led to open conversations on options around sharing theatre and outpatient capacity, working flexibly across organizations, developing a shared One Stop diagnostic service, streamlining multidisciplinary case discussions and incorporating genomic testing more effectively.

The complexity and the politics of the healthcare system at the time of study meant that relationships had to be built slowly and around the shared vision and system goals. In addition, it was important that the innovations produced value not only to the organization but to the system as a whole. This was a new shift in mindset from inward thinking and working in silos to outward thinking and working as a system.

Lesson 5—Peer influence and opinion leadership

Traditionally, clinicians have always based their clinical decision making on evidence-based medicine which includes primarily complex and lengthy randomized clinical trials. What the real-life case studies have demonstrated is the influential role of key opinion leaders in embedding best practice when the evidence-base is not as strong (Greszczuk et al. 2018). Key opinion leaders are usually credible individuals whose clinical and/or research work is well known to others is the field and are used to influence clinical practice (Flodgren et al. 2011).

Peer opinion leadership was key for the decision to adopt new clinical protocols and to redesign breast cancer pathways during the pandemic. Without the support of the peer community, which was strengthened, as a result of the pandemic, it would have been very difficult to adopt and diffuse new clinical practices as quickly as they have been.

Lesson 6—Clinical leader incentivisation and empowerment

It is evident from all three cases that enabled clinical leaders who are given the autonomy, space and power to innovate and transform clinical practice can be catalytical in the successful implementation of innovation. The opposite is also true of clinical leaders who are not engaged enough in the innovation process.

Clinical leader incentivisation can take various forms, including financial (external incentives) as well as non-financial or internal incentives (training, personal and professional development, time and space in job plan for innovation, ownership of projects, promotion). The question of 'what's in it for me' has come up many times and throughout all cases.

In case 3, the initiatives proposed for the Trust were backed up by the Integrated Care System which had already worked through the benefit realisation plan. This enabled a consistent and clear message being communicated top down and bottom up. In addition, the presence of a strong meso-level leadership ensured that the top-down strategy was implemented and there was a culture of shared vision and followship overcoming any strong clinician resistance. The engagement of doctor champions ensured that doctor concerns were addressed along the way (Boonstra et al. 2014). Clinical leaders of all disciplines could visualize and also verbalize the benefits of the new strategic direction for them, their patients and the communities they serve, which kept their internal motivation high at all times.

In case 1, the evaluation strategy of the project was very comprehensive and included amongst all aspects, staff and end user experience, usability and acceptability of the new technology, work efficiencies and quality of care. However, the business case and stakeholder presentations and engagement sessions focused more on the ROI (return on investment) aspect rather than the QI (quality improvement) aspect. In large digital transformation projects, it is important to talk about the short-term improvements which are usually quick wins on quality and safety, rather than the cost savings (ROI) which are more long-term (Wachter 2016). The lack of clinical leader engagement and involvement in the case 1 met with resistance from the doctor front, as they could not see 'what was in it for them'. In addition, the lack of Trust's commitment to innovation meant that the necessary extra resources (time, space, funding, training) for clinical leaders to be involved with innovation, were unavailable. As a result, clinical leaders saw the project more as a chore which conflicted with the day-to-day operational challenges rather than an exciting new model of care to work on.

Case 2 specific evaluation criteria were used to engage the clinical leaders which included improvements in the access, quality and efficiency of services. The detailed measurement of those benefits though came later in the process and after 12 months, as the initial focus of the organization was on the financial evaluation of the transformation program early on in the process. The latter attracted some but not the majority of clinical leaders who were more focused on the quality outcomes for their patients. It was clear though that the improvement of those quality parameters would help the organization deliver a wider engagement activity internally and externally, which would improve the bottom line in the long-term.

References

Boonstra A, Versluis A, Vos JFJ (2014) Implementing electronic health records in hospitals: a systematic literature review. BMC Health Serv Res 14:370

Brown BB et al (2014) Clinician-led improvement in cancer care (CLICC), testing a multifaceted implementation strategy to increase evidence-based prostate cancer care: phased randomised controlled trial—Study protocol. Implement Sci 2014(9):64

Corrigan P, Craig G et al (2013) People powered commissioning. Nesta

Flodgren G, Parmelli E, Doumit G et al (2011) Local opinion leaders: effects on professional practice and health care outcomes. Cochrane Database Syst Rev CD000125

Greszczuk C, Mughal F, Mathew R, Rashid A (2018) Peer influence as a drive of technological innovation in the UK National Health Service: a qualitative study of clinicians' experiences and attitudes. BMJ Innov 4:68–74

Kremer H, Villamor I, Aguinis H (2019) Innovation leadership: best-practice recommendations for promoting employee creativity, voice, and knowledge sharing. Bus Horiz 62:65–72

Kuratko DF, Hornsby JS, Covin JG (2014) Diagnosing a firm's internal environment for corporate entrepreneurship. Bus Horiz 57:37–47

NHS Confederation (2021) Integration and innovation: working together to improve health and social care for all

Powell A, Davies H (2016) Managing doctors, Doctors managing. Nuffield Trust

Schoenfeldt LF, Jansen KJ (1997) Methodological requirements for studying creativity in organizations. J Creat Behav 31(1):73–90

Wachter RM (2016) Making IT work: harnessing the power of health IT to improve care in England. National Advisory Group on Health IT in England

7

A Contemporary Framework of Leadership in Innovation

Abstract The three case studies have demonstrated that there are some key ingredients in making healthcare innovation adoption, diffusion and implementation a success, based on individual and organizational leadership behaviours. In the last case study, the proposed model of innovation was tested and further lessons learned were derived which have helped to refine and finalise the model. Those are summarised in the next section.

7.1 Leadership Lessons for Innovation Success

Contemporary healthcare organizations are in a state of innovation alertness and the success in their innovation journey, depend on the internal organizational readiness and agency of innovation as well as the external environment. The leadership lessons learned through the three organizational journeys of innovation, have led to the following conclusions which have informed the final model of leadership in innovation.

- *Strong leadership at system level and not just at organizational level* is key to healthcare innovation success. This would require close working between commissioners of healthcare services and patients (end users of services), primary and secondary care providers, the voluntary and private sectors, academia and the industry, in order to agree on commissioning services that really matter to patients. Some recent popular examples of such services include the remote monitoring of patients by clinical teams using digital technology, digital patient self-management tools for chronic conditions, as well as the expansion of social prescribing. What's common to all those services is the fact that they are all community—based services and services closer to patient homes which represents a value-adding societal benefit.
- *Key opinion leaders (KOLs)* are the legitimate and respected clinical representatives, who need to work together with top managers and commissioners to embed the clinical evidence for innovation into healthcare organizations. Non-peer KOLs can work collaboratively with peer KOLs to inspire ideation, present the evidence and their experience, as well as assign innovation champions to support innovation diffusion and implementation. Early involvement of KOLs is key at the ideation and adoption stage of innovation. A supportive peer community is also key to innovation diffusion, which begins with a well led clinical engagement strategy based on shared vision and purpose. Power differences between peers may be mitigated through the inclusion of non-peer KOLs to influence the peer community.

- *Meso-level clinical leadership* working collaboratively with the operational management team can bridge the gap between executive sponsors, commissioners and front-line clinicians. In addition, the leadership of the meso-level leader can work as an agent for change, spearheading innovation potential and working closer with the operational management team to create innovation capabilities within healthcare organizations. The meso-level clinical leadership plays a key role in bridging the gap between operational delivery and entrepreneurship.
- *Innovations in healthcare should benefit the society as a whole* and not just individual patients, based on a shared vision and goals that encompasses the whole integrated care system. The complexity and uncertainties of the current healthcare system means that stakeholder relationships have to be built slowly and around the shared vision and system goals. It is important that healthcare innovations produce value not only for individual organizations but also for the system and society as a whole. This represents a new shift in mindset from inward organizational thinking and working in silos to outward thinking and working as a system.
- *Clinician incentivization is critical* in the innovation process in order for them to engage consistently throughout the process. No matter how small or large scaled the innovation process is, clinicians are driven by a strong sense of purpose and meaning in their activities which more often than not involves a better quality of care for their patients. A robust benefit analysis with a clear benefit evaluation and communication plan that starts early in the innovation process (ideation and adoption stage), can help sustain clinician interest and engagement. Matrix working in a multidisciplinary approach between clinicians, managers, executives

within an organization and across clinical networks creates a sense of purpose and cultivates compassionate leadership. Time and space to think and innovate within organizations can incentivize clinicians to embark into innovation. Others will be incentivized by the prospect of idea commercialization resulting in revenue acquisition and/or professional accreditation and promotion. The 'what's in it for me' has to be well thought through for key stakeholders involved in small or large scale innovation.

- What has been evident during the COVID pandemic, is that the UK healthcare system cannot work on its own and without partnering with other providers including the private sector. *Partnerships are essential throughout all stages of innovation.* We need to do something differently moving into the future as an NHS because patients are expecting more responsive services and persistent high-quality services that can be accessed on demand, without queues and waiting times. To be able to achieve this, providers may need to combine forces so that they offer a truly personalized care and patient experience.
- *Top-down directional support* (ICS leaders, commissioners, executives with power to commission innovation) is key in setting the vision and purpose of the innovation and transformation strategy. This is particularly important in the early (adoption) and late stages of innovation (sustainability), when there is a need for low resistance to adoption and leveraging of powerful networks, respectively. A flexible top-down and bottom-up approach in leadership is needed at the diffusion and implementation stage of innovation, which requires clinician engagement and investment (buy-in) in the innovation.

7.2 Final Model for Leadership in Innovation Success

Putting the lessons learned together from all case studies, the proposed leadership in innovation model is presented in Fig. 7.1.

The innovation model of the future for healthcare organizations, is a harmonious combination of top-down leadership and bottom-up agency in order to transform organizational processes and innovation behaviours.

Clinicians, managers, commissioners, patients and the industry should work closely together to prioritize and work out innovative solutions to healthcare problems.

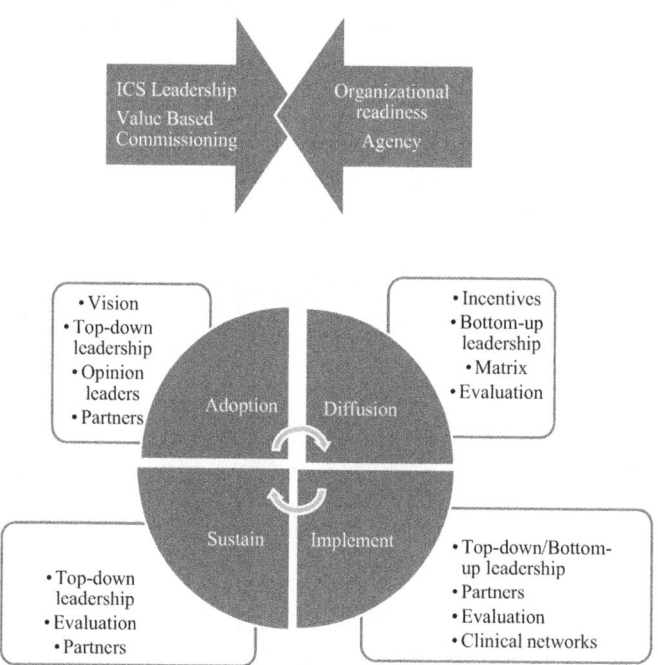

Fig. 7.1 Model of leadership in innovation success©

Organizations and systems who embark into their innovation and transformation journeys will benefit from our model for leadership in innovation.

Our model can be used as the framework for healthcare organizations to build their innovation and transformation strategy, whether this involves small or large-scale change. The digital innovation in case 1 involved a small scale change involving one particular clinical area in an organization, but with the potential to spread and scale up across other clinical areas. The innovation program in case 2 involved a large-scale change and a service transformation strategy which could be scaled in other markets where the group operated. Finally, the transformation program in case 3 involved a large-scale change at the organizational and healthcare system level. Leadership enablers needed to flex according to the stage of innovation in all three cases and the minimum ingredients, as described in the model, needed to be present so as to maximize chances of innovation success.

Appendix A: Methodology

Case studying is a methodology that when properly carried out, provides an in-depth understanding of certain phenomena such as healthcare innovation adoption and diffusion. In this book, the problem is well-defined and it is about the role of leadership in the success of innovation adoption, diffusion and implementation, within complex healthcare organizations.

The in-depth case studies are most suited to address the 'why' and 'how', what works and what doesn't, provide an explanatory analysis and also help with the induction of new models for leadership in innovation. The ethnographic approach taken by the innovator across the three case studies helped to generate rich data to explain enablers and barriers to innovation, as the innovator was fully immersed in the studied environments. It also enabled comparison between different innovation environments.

The choice of three different and complex innovation case studies was deliberate as they were written at realtime and as innovation processes unfolded. As such, the innovation outcomes are real and the description of success and failure contributory factors is accurate, through the numerous observations, discussions and participant interviews. Successful and failed innovation processes have been observed and evaluated in order to offer the reader a realistic perspective and useful learnings from all of them.

The inclusion of an NHS organization, studied at different points of time, has demonstrated the impact of the different politico-economical and social influences in the process of innovation. The opportunity to study an organization pre-pandemic (case 1) and in the context of a global pandemic (case 3), was key in capturing the healthcare system transformation component of innovation and leadership. The pandemic has spearheaded innovation acceleration across the UK and globally and emphasized the importance of certain critical success factors for innovation, such as the role of early top-down and visionary leadership, the early commissioner involvement in the innovation process, and the role of local (matrix working), regional (integrated care systems) and national partnerships (clinical networks and partnerships). The large shift in the organizational readiness for innovation for this organization was triggered by the learnings of the failed innovation (case 1), the pandemic spearheading innovation and change and the introduction of integrated care systems.

The study of a private healthcare organization demonstrated that innovation processes are similar in public and private organizations. The impact of top-down visionary leaders, the role of peer and non-peer key opinion leadership, the importance of the clinician agent of innovation who sits between executive sponsorship and front-line clinicians and the requirement for partner engagement, are key commonalities. What is different in the commercial sector is the role of commissioning, the organizational readiness for innovation and the internal resources and capabilities which are stronger in entrepreneurial commercial organizations than the public ones.

Epilogue

The National Health Service is facing significant demand and capacity challenges due to the ageing population and the higher cost of chronic illness (cardiovascular disease, diabetes, stroke and cancer), which is becoming more prevalent. The cost of chronic illness and ageing is due to expensive treatments, high emergency hospital admission rates, long length of hospital stays and increasing mental health costs. The financial sustainability of the NHS depends on a clear shared vision for innovation amongst all stakeholders, including commissioners, patients and healthcare professionals. By engaging in innovation, the NHS can continue to attract an innovative and highly talented workforce who can implement innovation to achieve cost efficiencies and better models of care.

Integrated Care Systems (ICSs) are well placed to promote innovation including digital transformation and to drive health improvements at population level.

Although the ICS leadership structure has not yet been organised fully, system leaders have set a rich innovation agenda for the next few years. Inevitably, the delivery of the innovation outcomes will need dedicated clinicians working in positions of power and decision-making. A number of new clinical leadership roles are being created to engage the clinical community as a result. The clinician of the future will have a diverse role portfolio compared to what front-line clinician have at present, which is purely service provision. This will require leadership training that starts earlier in the clinician educational curriculum, even at the undergraduate stage and should be supplemented with postgraduate and on-the-job leadership training.

Healthcare organizations currently exist in a state of 'innovation alertness' driven by consumer demand and provider competition. Investing in innovation could result in new, patient-centred and more efficient services. The key to achieving the vision for innovation is a united healthcare system, organizational as well as local clinical leadership. Leadership should be an agile combination of top-down and bottom-up approach, driving clinician and patient engagement. Healthcare professionals should be more involved in leadership and occupy more positions of power, so that they can act as expert agents of change.

The future NHS should be a clinically led healthcare system.

The proposed innovation model is applicable to any healthcare organization who is embarking into a journey of innovation and transformation. The book offers useful insights into the process of innovation within healthcare organizations as well as the leadership enablers for making innovation adoption, diffusion and implementation, a success.

Made in the USA
Monee, IL
03 May 2026